HAPPY
WITH BABY

To Rick, Hugh, and Lena, without whom the abundance of love, endless laughter, great patience - let alone this book - would be made been possible. I love the three of you always and forever.

And to all of the couples who have sat across from me in my office, in workshops, and via Zoom, shared their hearts and stories with me, and who have trusted me in the past and present with their relationships and the love that they have for each other - thank you for teaching me, guiding me, and co-creating supports and tried and true techniques for better living and loving with me.

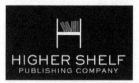

Contact information for Higher Shelf Publishing Company–
highershelfpublishing.com

ISBN: 978-1-7350466-0-0 (print)
ISBN: 978-1-7350466-1-7 (ebook)

Ordering Information:
Special discounts are available on quantity purchases by corporations, associations, and others. For details, contact admin@happywithbaby.com, www.happywithbaby.com, 916-718-9501

Table of Contents

HAPPY WITH BABY

Essential Relationship Advice When Partners Become Parents

Catherine O'Brien
with Rick Heyer

Introduction

You will love your child more than you ever thought possible, but there will come a time (if there hasn't already) when you will wonder if they will always need you 23 hours and 39 minutes every day. You love your partner, with whom you are sharing this great gift, but where are they hiding? Didn't they say they'd be gone only a minute and now five hours later, you've changed 111 diapers? Wouldn't you know it, you had a baby and *then* the arguments started.

On top of that, you worry and question everything you do with your baby: if I feed them the wrong brand of applesauce, will they still be able to get into a good college?

You weren't expecting this—what gives?

While you're worrying about your child, may I take a minute to worry about you and your significant other? Because almost 70 percent of couples say their marriage struggled in the first three years of their child's life[1]. That's right, 70 percent.

Years from now, someone may ask you about your greatest accomplishments in life. It's likely that on the list will be your wonderful child or children. You may be asked what gives you the most happiness and you may respond the same way.

But during your child's first year, that response won't come easily. Let me put your mind at ease: Your kids are going to turn out amazing. You will make some mistakes that grandparents will point out to you. (These are your parents, who somehow have no memory of how they raised you.) Not to mention, random people at the supermarket.

There will be ups and downs, but each year raising your child will get easier (and maybe more difficult in other ways). But if you and your significant other don't take the time to ask yourself some questions and work together every day, you could build up a wall of resentment that could linger for years in your relationship.

Because another great accomplishment you'll be just as proud of is how strong your relationship is and how, by working together, you headed off any problems you might have had. It's important to do this now because when your children are grown, your partner is who you will be spending 23 hours and 39 minutes with every day.

How Do I Know?

As a Licensed Marriage and Family Therapist for almost 20 years, I have conducted thousands of counseling sessions with both individuals and couples on how to meet the challenges in their lives. Over the last decade, I've concentrated on working with new and expecting parents on the challenges they face when they bring home a new baby.

My desire to help new parents came out of feeling completely unprepared for the impact that bringing home our first baby would have on my relationship with my husband. Through my own struggles, I began compiling all the things I wished I'd known. That is how I developed my first workshop, "Mine, Yours,

Ours: Relationship Survival Guide to Baby's 1st Year." One of the biggest rewards of that experience has been the perspective of my husband, Rick, as he began co-facilitating the workshop with me. Feedback from our workshop attendees is always well-received because of the perspectives of both parents. We've included these voices, these perspectives for that very same reason. Not only are two parents dealing with the changes associated with having a newborn but also each person comes with their own perspective.

Throughout this book, you will meet couples who will share frustrating experiences you might relate to as well as solutions they found beneficial.

I've divided the book into three sections; these are Part I: Taking Care of Yourself, Part II: Taking Care of Your Relationship, and Part III: Taking Care of Baby. I purposely start with taking care of yourself because this is often where new parents struggle the most in the first year of their baby's life. Believe it or not, you can get so focused on making sure your baby's needs are met that you completely forget to take care of yourself. Just as when flying on an airplane, you must put on your own oxygen mask before you can help someone else. Or put another way, you can't pour from an empty cup. Equally important, you can assume that your partner is taking care of himself or herself and forget to make time to nurture the relationship.

I've worked with parents across the spectrum: queer, married, unmarried, co-habitating, co-parenting.[2] I've worked with groups of parents, many of them struggling with how to cope with the newness of bringing home a baby and the impact on their family, their relationship. I've also mentored other therapists who are working with new parents. Through the years, I've compiled a list of solutions I have researched or have received from parents in my practice or who have attended my workshops.

In the end, my most important attribute for helping new parents is how I sucked at being a new mom and a co-parent. At least I did until I got help from people I respect. They helped me see how my expectations of motherhood set me up for feelings of failure. In this book, Rick and I are going to show you how to overcome your own struggle and share with you how others just like you learned to deal with theirs.

Clearly, the first few years are tougher than most, but you're not shipwrecked on an island. You have each other and the many couples who in this book will share secrets to making your life easier and better.

Most of your child's early years will be wonderful, but we'll help make the hard parts easier so that your relationship stays as strong as your love for your baby.

Disclaimer: Parenthood is messy and so are relationships. The case studies in the book are based on real couples. The names and some facts have been changed.

ENDNOTES

1   Alison F Shapiro, et al., "Effects on Marriage of a Psycho-Communicative-Educational Intervention With Couples Undergoing the Transition to Parenthood, Evaluation at 1-Year Post Intervention," *The Journal of Family Communication* 5, no. 1 (2005): 1-24, https://doi.org/10.1207/s15327698jfc0501_1.

2   A note about gender: In this book, as in my practice, I always strive to be inclusive and sensitive to the ways that gender and identity play into our experiences as parents and as human beings. I also hope to make this book as clear and easy to read as possible. If you, dear reader, were sitting across from me in my office, I would ask how you identify as a person and as a parent and which are your preferred pronouns so I could honor the language that most resonates with you. Because that isn't possible in this format, these are the pronouns I am using for clarity's sake: *she/her/hers* to refer to mothers and *he/him* to refer to fathers/partners.

Part I:
Taking Care of Yourself

CHAPTER 1

The New Parent Quick-Start Guide

Usually when you bring home something new, it comes with a manual or a quick-start guide. Chances are, you got one for your lawnmower, DVD player, or La-Z-Boy recliner. But with your new baby, what did you get? Nothing. Sure, you have a few baby books that say what the baby needs but not who's supposed to do what or when.

We hear it from new parents all the time: No one ever told them that it was going to be this hard. I'm not sure how we end up feeling so ill-prepared. As a society, we are really good at planning for a big day. We plan great birthday parties and great weddings. We spend so much time preparing all the details for these special days—the flowers, color of balloons, type of cake, choice of clothing—everything. But what about what happens after?

The same goes for having a baby. There's so much prep for the actual "event." You take classes that discuss how you should prepare your birth plan, how you should breathe, what to expect from the transitions in early and active labor. You tour the hospital or birth center or make preparations to have your baby at home; you discuss who you want (or don't want) to be in the room. But what happens after? What happens when you bring the baby home?

Maybe we'd have never gone through with it if we'd had any idea how things were going to go. We were truly unprepared for the impact this tiny little human would have on our lives. Oh, how naive we were.

Because of our own struggles, Rick and I want other couples to avoid being so blindsided. We want parents to feel more prepared, to get some idea of what to expect and a bit of a game plan on how to go about it. Of course, as with any game plan, adjustments will be made. But a plan is better than no plan.

You will have to keep checking in with each other to make sure that everything is going as best as can be expected. Regular check-ins are highly encouraged.

Here, I've sketched out some tips when bringing home baby. I'll talk about these in more detail, but this list will get you started, and you can reference it anytime for a quick reminder.

- **Provide support.** Offer each other support and encouragement. Having a new baby is a new experience for both of you. It can be challenging to try and figure out how to meet the needs of your precious little one. It is important to be able to support each other and acknowledge that you are both in this together, as a team. If one of you is feeling discouraged or overwhelmed, make sure to provide encouraging words and support.

- **Check in daily.** Make time to check in with each other every day. One of the biggest complaints that Rick and I hear from couples is they never communicate anymore. When you have children, it takes more effort to make time for each other, so get in a habit of taking 10 to 15 minutes each day to talk about how each of you is doing.

- **Monitor your mental health.** Make sure that you address with your partner how you are coping emotionally. The number one complication of childbirth is a postpartum mood or anxiety disorder.[3] Up to 20 percent of new mothers[4] experience this, and up to 10 percent of new fathers.[5] Know the risk factors and signs to look for because the earlier it is treated (and it is treatable), the better off the family as a whole will be. Ask for help! (See Chapter 2 for details.)

- **Sleep.** Do take any and all opportunities to get some ZZZs. Everything seems worse when you are not getting enough sleep. Reports show that new parents lose anywhere from over 500 hours[6] to more than 1000 hours[7] of sleep in their child's first year of life. If you have friends or family members willing to watch your child so that you can get some REM sleep, take them up on the offer. No awards are given out to parents who never take any help. It does take a village!

- **Evaluate your expectations.** Sometimes what we expect to happen, dream of happening, or wish to have happened gets in the way of what *really* happens and that affects how we are experiencing what is happening. Your baby will not do what you want them to do. Chances are, your birth experience will not be how it was "supposed to be," your baby won't sleep how and when you want them to, and quite possibly the feeding process won't be as natural as it seems it should be. But that can also be the beauty of parenting because having children makes us grow in ways we never expected.

- **Don't keep score.** There is no fair way to evaluate who is doing more or who is doing it better. If you are feeling overwhelmed, talk with your partner. Chances are very high that they are feeling the same way.

- **Remember that nothing lasts forever.** This "new baby" time is a short period in your child's life. You will be overwhelmed, you will be tired, you will ask yourself what the hell you got yourself into. Relax. This time won't last forever, things will change, and what is difficult now will get easier.

- **Honor each other's learning curve.** All new parents will have a learning curve —some things will be easier for you and some will be easier for your partner. Give each other a chance to figure things out. Don't micromanage how each of you does things.

- **Present a united front.** Maintain a united front with your partner. This is good practice when dealing with your parents or in-laws and will be good practice for when your baby is older and starts having an opinion about things.

- **Keep your perspective.** Take everything you hear from those around you with a grain of salt. They mean well but sometimes your family and friends say things that can feel upsetting and hurtful, maybe because you're tired and already doubting yourself. Remember, just because someone advises or recommends something does not mean it is the right thing for you and your family.

- **Say "I love you."** This can get forgotten, but please don't neglect to tell each other every day that you love each other. It is so easy to let the relationship slide when you have a new child because all your focus shifts to the baby. You are tired and have limited energy. However, it is critical that your partner knows they are still important to you.

- **Schedule a date night.** Make sure to "date" each other at least once a week, whether that means taking a walk with the baby in a stroller, playing a game together while the baby sleeps, or even going out to lunch or dinner.

If you're reading this list and are unsure how you can make it work with your tiny new human, don't worry, we have lots of ideas and suggestions—keep reading. Take what is helpful. Try something new. If it doesn't work, tweak it for *your* family or try something else. But don't give up. Things get better the more you work together.

THINGS THAT CHANGE

- Sleep patterns
- Availability of time
- Financial support for family
- Cost of childcare
- Work situation/status
- Financial preparation for child's schooling
- Purchase of baby clothes
- Time spent together as a couple
- Communication as a couple
- Concern about partner's needs
- Decline in sexual interest
- Couple's disagreements about roles
- Loss (or confusion) of identity
- Loss of free time for self and social activities
- Personal doubts about competence or skills as a parent
- Diaper changing
- Individual stress about roles and responsibilities
- Decisions about childcare
- Unhappiness with personal appearance/change in body shape
- Decreased time for TV watching
- Anxiety about child's well-being
- Overstimulation of child
- Nutritional needs of child
- Increased chores and housework
- Cleanliness of home
- Recovery from labor and delivery
- Unpredictable shifts in mood and anxiety
- Relationships with parents, in-laws, and other family members
- Relationships with friends

THREE DAILY QUESTIONS

These three questions not only form the final part of our quick-start guide but also provide the structure for this entire book. We'll be discussing them in depth as you read along but keep them in mind as you begin this journey. And consider them on a daily basis. They are easy to ask but very often hard to answer. Be encouraged that the more you ask them, the easier they will be to answer. Think of a daily consideration of them as self-care for your entire family unit.

1. What will you do to take care of and reconnect with yourself?

2. What will you do to support and connect with your partner?

3. What will you do to nurture and connect with your baby?

The great thing about these questions is that as your baby grows, they can be changed and added to. It is important to continue to assess the needs of your family and to talk with your partner about what you need from each other to continue to be—happy with baby.

RICK'S TAKE

The moment I knew that I was not the Superdad I had hoped to be came one morning in our son's first year. That's when I realized I was keeping score of how much I was doing to take care of the baby—compared with how much Catherine was doing. It was 3:30 a.m.; the baby was crying and Catherine was still lying in bed. I was convinced that Catherine's score was woefully lower than mine and that it was her turn to attend to the baby. I conveyed that and she conveyed right back to me her belief I was, in fact, full of shit.

Later that day we talked. It turned out that we both were seeing only what we were doing to take care of the baby and failing to appreciate the contribution of the other. If we had not had that discussion, the toxic habit of keeping score would have continued and festered. Talking honestly that day allowed us both to express how tired we were and how frustrated we were feeling. It also allowed us to appreciate that we were both feeling the same frustrations. We took from that conversation a promise to stop keeping score because we realized how poisonous it was to our relationship.

ENDNOTES

3   Bradley N. Gaynes et al., "Perinatal Depression: Prevalence, Screening Accuracy, and Screening Outcomes," *Evidence Report/Technology Assessments*, no. 119 (2005): 1-8, https://doi.org/10.1037/e439372005-001.

4   Nicole Fairbrother et al., "Depression and Anxiety During the Perinatal Period," *BMC Psychiatry* 15, no. 206 (Aug 2015): https://doi.org/10.1186/s12888-015-0526-6.

5   James F. Paulson et al., "Prenatal and Postpartum Depression in Fathers and Its Association With Maternal Depression: A Meta-Analysis," *JAMA* 303, no.19 (May 2010): https://doi.org/10.1001/jama.2010.605.

6   Erika W. Hagen et al., "The Sleep-Time Cost of Parenting: Sleep Duration and Sleepiness Among Employed Parents in the Wisconsin Sleep Cohort Study," *American Journal of Epidemiology* 177, no. 5 (March 2013): 394–401, https://doi.org/10.1093/aje/kws246.

7   Heather Marcoux, "New parents lose 44 days of sleep during the first year of baby's life," Motherly.com, accessed June 5, 2020, https://www.mother.ly/news/sleep-1.

CHAPTER 2

PMAD: The Sneaky Thief of New Baby Joy

The number one complication of childbirth is a postpartum mood or anxiety disorder (PMAD)[8]. Up to 20 percent of women experience this, and up to 10 percent of their partners. Your partner's risk goes up to 50 percent if mom is experiencing a mood disorder. That is why we start here—with one particularly challenging situation.[9]

STEVEN AND AVA'S STORY
Steven reached out to me shortly after the birth of his and his wife Ava's first child. He expressed concerns about Ava's possible symptoms of postpartum depression and anxiety. Moreover, he emphasized that she wasn't open to coming to therapy. He felt that she needed help and he wasn't sure what to do. He shared that she was in a really negative place. He sensed a lot of unresolved conflict and was seeing a lot of anger.

Since Ava wasn't in a place to start therapy, Steven started coming to see me alone so that he could figure out how to support her and understand how to best help her.

STEVEN'S PERSPECTIVE

I don't know what's going on with Ava. She hasn't been herself. I know that she was looking forward to going back to work but it seems to have added so much more stress. I feel like every time I say something to her, she blows up at me. I constantly feel like I'm walking on eggshells. I wish she knew that I only want to help her. It seems like we'll get into the groove, carry on like real people, but then the baby will have a few bad nights that keep us up and we seem to completely fall apart. I don't dare say I wish we hadn't had a baby but it makes me wonder if it's ever going to feel normal again.

What I really wish is that she'd accept the support being offered or take a break instead of feeling like she has to do everything. But every time I remotely suggest it, she reacts as if I'm making her feel like a less-than-perfect mom. I don't want her to think that I think she is crazy.

A big part of our therapy sessions was for Steven to be able to understand what Ava was feeling. He came to therapy believing that her experiences and feelings were not normal. He accepted that some negative emotions and thoughts were common, but he struggled to grasp the reality of postpartum depression and anxiety for new moms.

I educated him in what PMADs are and how they can manifest differently for different moms. I also counseled him in how to have discussions with Ava about getting the support she very much needed and deserved.

Sometimes new moms feel indifferent or they feel guilty because they don't have the sense of connection with their baby they think that they're supposed to have. Maybe they feel depressed or anxious as well as detached from their child. It may not feel safe to share these thoughts and feelings out of concern that you'll be perceived as a bad mom, but it's even more important to have a support system in place when you're feeling low.

It's important for you to know that first and foremost, PMADs are highly treatable. There's no reason that you can't feel much,

much better soon. Second, there's absolutely nothing to be embarrassed or ashamed about; you just need to find the right help. Talk with your obstetrician or find a therapist who specializes in treating PMADs. Visit postpartum.net for resources in your area.

After a while, when Ava started feeling a little bit better, she was able to get therapy on her own. Eventually, she attended a few couple's sessions with Steven to address and repair some of the damage to their relationship.

AVA'S SITUATION

Now that her maternity leave was coming to an end, Ava had begun doubting herself more than ever. She wanted to go back to work, but she was already so exhausted and irritated from the baby refusing to sleep more than three hours in a row that she didn't know how on earth she'd cope. It had been a bad couple of nights with little sleep, but for Ava, it felt like she hadn't slept in months. Everything agitated her: the sound of Steven's breathing, the way the dishwasher left the glassware all spotty, the nonstop fussing when she tried to nurse.

She was looking forward to going back to work to have a break from the baby, which made her feel 10 times more guilty. She had to be the worst mom on the planet. She'd even begun to doubt her motives for getting pregnant in the first place.

It had seemed like such a great idea at the time, getting pregnant. She'd always wanted children and she knew that Steven would make a wonderful father. But now everything seemed so hard and she felt trapped in a daily grind of poop, spit up, and dirty laundry. How come no one had told her it would be this hard? Why didn't anyone else seem to be struggling like she was? How could Steven be the same happy-go-lucky guy he'd always been? Clearly, she wasn't cut out to be a mother. She fantasized about running away to a little beach town where she could work in a used bookstore.

This line of thinking must mean that she was a monster. She was feeling super depressed, super anxious, and super guilty, all rolled into one. She wanted to climb out of her own skin. What was wrong with her, she wondered.

She'd read about postpartum depression more than once, but really, if push came to shove, she felt more anxious than depressed most of the time. So, it couldn't be that. And God forbid she tell people how she was *really* feeling, most of all Steven. The last thing she needed was for him to be dismissive of her feelings or worse feel overly concerned and think she was a terrible mother and leave with the baby.

When Ava last told Steven how tired she was, he just said, "Me too." She asked him if having a baby was harder than he'd thought it would be and he said no, he knew it would be hard. That's what he'd signed up for. The only thing that conversation served to do was leave her feeling invalidated and like an idiot for not realizing any of this reality stuff before.

Why did he have to be so damn smug? She accused Steven of having it easy because he didn't have to do all the work. He got to go off to his workplace and have a good time doing what he was good at. She was the one who was left picking up the slack. Once she went back to work, it would only get worse.

In her less-anxious moments, Ava knew that she was projecting all her doubts and frustrations onto Steven, accusing him of wishing the baby had never been born. He of course got defensive. From the perplexed look on his face, she could tell that he had no idea where she had come up with such things.

Ava hated being irrational. There had to be a root cause.

What is a PMAD?
Being diagnosed with a PMAD is *not* a life sentence. There are many helpful treatment options. The sooner you seek help, the sooner you can start feeling better. Please don't wait to ask for help.

You are not a monster if you suffer from a PMAD, even though you may feel like one. There are a number of contributing factors that make one woman more susceptible than others, many of which should allow you to feel less guilty.

POSTPARTUM MOOD AND ANXIETY DISORDER (PMAD) RISK FACTORS[10]

- Family history of PMADs
- Family history of mood or anxiety disorders
- Stressors, e.g., a move, divorce, death, financial troubles
- Stressful relationship with significant other
- Lack of support
- Complications during pregnancy
- Traumatic labor and delivery
- Mother of multiples
- Baby or babies in NICU
- Thyroid imbalance
- Vitamin D deficiency[11]
- History of miscarriage[12]
- Unplanned pregnancy[13]
- Complications with breastfeeding[14]
- "Type A" personality
- High expectations of motherhood
- Supermom syndrome[15]
- Fussy, colicky, high-needs baby[16]

PMADs often get confused with or chalked up to having a bad day. A few nights without sleep, a change in schedule, a fight with your partner can all contribute to a sense of malaise. How do you know if you're just having a bad couple of days or if you're the one in five[17] moms experiencing a PMAD?

SYMPTOMS CHECKLIST

If you experience any of the following symptoms **for two weeks or more** during your pregnancy (yes, you can even experience these symptoms while you are pregnant) or within a year after your child's birth, please contact your doctor or visit postpartum.net for resources and support in your area:

- Feeling sad or a lack of joy or pleasure
- Feeling a lack of interest in your child(ren), your usual activities, or interacting with others
- Feeling irritable, agitated, or angry with those around you or with circumstances
- Having problems eating or sleeping (either too much or not enough)
- Crying often or most of the time
- Blaming yourself unnecessarily or feeling very guilty
- Feeling hopeless, helpless, or worthless
- Having thoughts of or worries about harming yourself or your child(ren)[18]
- Feeling anxious, worried, scared, tense, or panicky without good reason[19]
- Not looking forward to things with enjoyment
- Having recurrent nightmares or reliving past traumatic events[20]
- Counting, checking, cleaning, or other repetitive behaviors
- Having intrusive, repetitive, or upsetting thoughts that you can't get out of your mind[21]

- Seeing, hearing, or feeling things that others do not
- Experiencing paranoia[22]

Please know that pregnancy and postpartum depression and anxiety symptoms are different for every woman—and so are the signs that indicate the need for treatment.

Many women experience some mild mood changes during or after the birth of a child. With proper care and support, you can prevent a worsening of these symptoms and that you can fully recover. This is not your fault and there is no reason to continue to suffer!

PMAD Support System

Beyond getting professional treatment for a PMAD, you'll also want to create a support system. It's vital to have some help. (See Chapter 18 for tips on developing a community of support.)

Make a list of people who can support you, stay with you, and offer you a hand or an ear:

- Grandparents
- Friends
- Postpartum doula
- Night nurse
- Other: _____

Also make an emergency contact list:

- ER
- Primary care physician
- Crisis nursery

How to Help a Partner with a PMAD

Like Steven, many partners of moms suffering with a PMAD do

not know how to help. Fortunately, there are some simple ways for a partner to be supportive, which will ease the stress for all involved.

- **Acknowledge that this is hard for her; validate her struggle.** Reassure her that just because she's having a difficult time doesn't make her a bad mom. Many moms are reluctant to get help because they fear that somehow they're failing as a mom or they're not a good mom or not meant to be a mom. So, acknowledge that it's hard. As with all new things, it takes time to adjust.

- **Reassure her; let her know that you're there for her.** Whether you're physically at home with her or just checking in with a call or text—even if you don't get a response every time—just keep letting her know, "Hey, I'm thinking about you. I'm here for you." If you can help her find a support group or a therapist or even line up friends and family to offer help, do so.

- **Love her unconditionally; let her know that you love her.** Remind her that she's a good person and that if she needs any support, anything, of course you're there.

RESOURCES FOR FURTHER (QUICK) READING
- *The Postpartum Husband: Practical Solutions for Living with Postpartum Depression* by Karen R. Kleiman (Xlibris Corporation, 2000). Check out Chapter 19 in particular for more of what to say to a mom who is struggling.
- *Beyond the Blues: Understanding and Treating Prenatal and Postpartum Depression & Anxiety* by Shoshana Bennett & Pec Indman (Moodswings Press, 2015). Check out Chapter 4 for more things to keep in mind and to say.

Ava and Steven are doing really well now. But there was quite a bit of time when things were really hard, and Steven wasn't sure how much longer he could go on with their little family in such a negative space. So, a big part of therapy was helping him to be able to understand what Ava was feeling and to offer support without minimizing her experiences and hurting her feelings. This seemed to help Ava open up more and be receptive to his support so that she was then able to get the therapy she needed.

Remember that you are not alone and that with help you can feel better.

ENDNOTES

8   Gaynes, "Perinatal Depression: Prevalence, Screening Accuracy, and Screening Outcomes."

9   Paulson, "Prenatal and Postpartum Depression in Fathers and Its Association With Maternal Depression: A Meta-Analysis."

10   "Depression During Pregnancy & Postpartum," Postpartum Support International, accessed June 9, 2020, https://www.postpartum.net/learn-more/depression-during-pregnancy-postpartum/.

11   Fariba Aghajafari et al., "Vitamin D Deficiency and Antenatal and Postpartum Depression: A Systematic Review," *Nutrients* 10, no. 4 (April 2018): 478. https://doi.org/10.3390/nu10040478.

12   Cara Bicking Kinsey et al., "Effect of Previous Miscarriage on Depressive Symptom s during Subsequent Pregnancy and Postpartum in the First Baby Study," Maternal and Child Health Journal 19, no. 2 (February 2015): 391-400, https://doi.org/10.1007/s10995-014-1521-0.

13   Nichole Fairbrother et al., "Perinatal anxiety disorder prevalence and incidence," *Journal of Affective Disorders*, no. 200 (August 2016): 148-55, https://doi.org/10.1016/j.jad.2015.12.082.

14   Samantha Metzer-Brody, "New Insights Into Perinatal Depression: Pathogenesis and Treatment During Pregnancy and Postpartum," Dialogues in Clinical Neuroscience 13, no. 1 (2011): 89-100.

15   Alessandro Ambrosini et al., "Early perinatal diagnosis of mothers at risk of developing post-partum depression – a concise guide for obstetricians, midwives, neonatologists and paediatricians," The Journal of Maternal-Fetal & Neonatal Medicine 25, no. 7 (2011): 1096-1101, https://doi.org/10.3109/14767058.2011.622011.

16   "Mothers of fussy babies at higher risk of depressive symptoms," ScienceDaily, published March 25, 2019, accessed June 9, 2020, https://www.sciencedaily.com/releases/2019/03/190325110321.htm.

17   Fairbrother et al., "Perinatal anxiety disorder prevalence and incidence."

18   "Depression During Pregnancy & Postpartum," Postpartum Support International.

19   "Anxiety During Pregnancy & Postpartum," Postpartum Support International, accessed June 9, 2020, https://www.postpartum.net/learn-more/anxiety-during-pregnancy-postpartum/.

20   "Postpartum Post-Traumatic Stress Disroder" Postpartum Support International, accessed June 30, 2020 https://www.postpartum.net/learn-more/postpartum-post-traumatic-stress-disorder/

21   "Pregnancy or Postpartum Obsessive Symptoms" Postpartum Support International, accessed June 30, 2020 https://www.postpartum.net/learn-more/pregnancy-or-postpartum-obsessive-symptoms/

22   "Postpartum Psychosis " Postpartum Support International, accessed June 30, 2020 https://www.postpartum.net/learn-more/postpartum-psychosis/

CHAPTER 3

Your Partner in Crime Needs Their Sidekick

Remember those three little words. You know what they are. And you need to say them every day. That's right, the three words are… "It's your turn!" No, actually, they are… "I love you!"

Some of you might be thinking that at the moment, you get more instant gratification out of "It's your turn!" But we're talking in the long run.

Tell your partner every day that you love them. It is so easy to let the relationship go when you have a new child because all your focus seems to shift to the ever-present, often-pressing needs of the baby. You are tired and have limited energy. You might even feel all "touched out" from the needs of the baby and making other expressions of affection is the last thing you feel like doing.

However, it is critical that your partner know they are still important to you and three little words are so easy to say. Deep down, don't you want to hear your partner say them to you?

You might say, "But, Catherine, words are cheap." That's fair. But there are other simple ways to say, "I love you."

One mom told me that while they were both in the weeds with new parenthood, she was feeling way too touched out to show much affection to her partner, let alone have sex with him. She said that every night, her partner would bring her a glass of water to keep beside her bed because he knew she would wake up thirsty from breastfeeding. And that spoke volumes.

We often hear from moms who express feeling all touched out from breastfeeding, leaving them with little desire for sex with their partner. Research shows that breastfeeding mothers may have a lower sex drive due to reduced estrogen levels,[23] making intercourse more uncomfortable. It's also possible that their higher levels of prolactin and oxytocin from breastfeeding and caring for their baby provide them with a sufficient sense of well-being and contentment so they feel less need to get affection from their partner.

KEVIN AND MANDY'S STORY

Kevin and Mandy were struggling in the intimacy department. Mandy shared that every time her partner, Kevin, would sit next to her on the couch, she would feel the pressure to have sex and it would increase tenfold if he started rubbing her shoulders. She was sure that meant he was going to want sex! If Kevin rubbed her shoulders, she interpreted that as a warm-up. She would do whatever it took to avoid being touched because if he started to touch her, she knew he was going to want to have sex.

The fact was, Kevin didn't want sex (well, he did want it) as much as he wanted to be close to Mandy. He was looking for ways to try and connect.

KEVIN'S PERSPECTIVE

I really miss spending time with Mandy. We used to do so much together, and now it feels like she is either spending time with the baby or finding ways to avoid me. I honestly would be happy some days just to be in the same room with her watching TV. I mean, don't get me wrong, if things led to more, I wouldn't turn her down. But I know that she's tired and that the baby makes so many demands on her physically. I just miss holding her.

MANDY'S PERSPECTIVE
I know that we need to spend "time together." I just really am not in the mood or the space to do anything. I feel like I just want to have my own time and space to not have to do anything for anyone.

We have heard it frequently, from a mother expressing annoyance, to her sensing a burden to provide something for her partner that she feels she has neither the energy, nor the desire to give.

Those times when you feel all touched out aren't just about not getting a break. They're about constant physical contact. Your baby is tugging at your clothes, your hair. Your baby is crying the second you set them down after being sound asleep in your arms. Your teething baby is needing constant soothing. Your fully weaned baby is still instinctively sticking her hand under your shirt to be breastfed.

Mom may be wondering, "When is my body going to belong to me again?"

Being the partner or a child of someone who doesn't want to be touched can feel awful. It feels like rejection. And being the person who causes that rejection can make you feel guilty and awful too.

The good news is that intimacy doesn't only mean sex and it isn't always about touch. It's about checking in and communicating with each other. Ultimately, it's about feeling a deeper connection with your partner. That's true intimacy. And you can still have that regardless of which phase of your parenting journey you're in.

So, when you're all touched out and have limited time and energy, how can you feel that connection to your partner? Here are a few really simple ways.

- **Intimacy is talking, and listening, to each other.** What do you need? How was your day? What happened? This is communication 101, right? But really, it makes all the difference. Being able to talk about the details of your day (however profound or mundane they might be) and to be truly heard with undivided attention...sometimes there isn't anything better. This is a great opportunity to ask for what you need. Do you need a break? Do you need to lie down alone for some free, untouched time? Do you need to get out into the fresh air for a 10-minute walk? To have your partner hear you and give you that space is such a loving gesture. It really makes all the difference.

- **Intimacy is doing the little things to help each other out.** You've probably seen images from those *Porn for Women* and *Porn for New Moms* books featuring attractive men doing things like housework or offering to take care of a crying baby. It's mostly tongue-in-cheek and a bit cliché but, as silly as it is, there is some truth to it. The point is, when our partner notices that the living room needs tidying or the dinner table needs clearing and takes it upon themselves to just get it done to help us out, we feel seen, validated, supported. It's such a subtle form of intimacy, but when our partner can say something like, "I know you hate cleaning up after dinner. Let's do it together and knock it out faster." Or, even better, "I've got the dishes. Why don't you go take that shower the baby didn't let you take earlier today? I'll bring you a hot towel from the dryer." I dare anyone to tell me that doesn't count as intimacy. I'll bet that your partner feels just as cared for when you make small gestures to make their day better too.

- **Intimacy is getting reacquainted with each other.** For some new parents—especially if one parent is a stay-at-home parent—having conversations that don't involve the baby or the kids can feel awkward or challenging. It can be tricky to find ways to relate to each other. It might even seem like you have to relearn how to socialize with grown-ups again. That's normal! Bringing a new baby into your home is a huge life change, and you have to be able to talk about what that actually looks and feels like for you. But if you find yourself stumped for a conversation starter, one thing that always feels productive is to learn something new about your partner or to share something new about yourself. If you need assistance with this, you can try table topic cards. Sometimes a free online quiz can be fun and enlightening; you can find all sorts of personality or relationship quizzes via a Google search. You're likely to learn something new about your partner and maybe even find yourself going off on conversational tangents of your own. That's great! Instead of defaulting to Netflix, why not have your at-home date with each other centered around getting reacquainted.

- **Intimacy is sometimes gestural.** Gestures are physical actions, but they don't have to mean sex or even touching. Curiously, sometimes people who feel touched out find that if they can be the one to give a hug (rather than waiting to receive one), it brings them back to a place of wanting to be touched again. If that's not going to happen today, why not try simple eye contact? Maybe that's a shared glance when your baby does something new or maybe it's something more prolonged and intentional. You get to decide here. I've had a mom tell me that the most intimate and romantic thing her partner did while their daughter was young was to reach across the bed at night to simply hold her hand after a rough day. She said she appreciated that he didn't inch closer to embrace her or to "make a move"—he just held her hand and continued to hold it until they fell asleep. I love that. It's a simple acknowledgement of, "Yes, this is hard, and yes, we both are exhausted, but I'm still here with you."

When parenthood puts you and your partner through the ringer, whether you're feeling touched out or not, you might want to give some of these suggestions a try. Maybe you're already doing one or two of them and didn't make the connection that this is also what intimacy looks like.

If passion and fireworks aren't happening right now, it's OK. It can take a while. That doesn't mean they won't ever come back. And in the meantime, you can keep that spark and connection going by coming back to the basics time and time again.

After recognizing that Kevin wasn't always trying to get lucky in the bedroom, Mandy started receiving what he was giving instead of putting a wall up to keep him out. She was able to see that he was rubbing her back simply because he wanted to be close to her. This made a huge difference in their interactions.

A lot of what Kevin and Mandy were doing showed that they loved each other. But still, remember to say it every day: "I love you…and now it's your turn."

YOU WANT ME TO GO ON A DATE?

Seems like a silly question, doesn't it? How do you even contemplate going on a date with your partner, the very person you find yourself irritated with nonstop? Especially when you have so much to do and when your life is promising to become even more difficult.

PUT IT ON THE CALENDAR

Get ready to pull out your calendar and start planning time to spend together right now, without exception. You may be thinking road trip with your posse. No, no, no.

Make sure to "date" each other at least once a week. This is a biggie! I know it can seem like an impossibility right now. You might even think that it's not necessary. After all, you're already committed, right? But loving relationships, like any other living, breathing thing, need nurturing to stay alive.

I, for one, can always tell when my husband and I are overdue for a date: I start to get annoyed by the trivial things I'd otherwise never notice. If I'm irritated that he forgot to blot the water splashes on the bathroom counter after brushing his teeth, I know we need to schedule a date, pronto.

When you have a baby at home, it can be helpful to reimagine what dating looks like to make it more achievable. It doesn't have to be dinner and dancing into the wee hours. Securing the childcare alone can make that kind of date seem out of reach.

Instead, maybe it's just going for a walk with the baby in a stroller, playing a game together while the baby sleeps, or even going out to lunch (with baby in tow). What matters is that your time is focused on each other and as close to uninterrupted as possible. Obviously, you can't do much about baby interrupting your time but you can put your phones away.

The great thing about babies when they're really small is that most of the time they'll do just fine in public spaces. They'll probably nap or stare at your face the whole time you're out for lunch, and they seem to tolerate the noise of a busy restaurant pretty well. This gets trickier when they're older, squirmier, and liable to make a mess. Not that you still can't go out with them—I'm actually all for it—but it may be more distracting for you when you're trying to keep your attention on your partner.

If securing a sitter is within your means, take advantage! Maybe your mother-in-law is dying for some one-on-one with her new grandbaby. Or maybe you can afford to hire help. That's great. We should all be so lucky.

So, if you have access to someone who is willing to take care of baby (whether paid or for free) and it works for you, *do it!* I don't mean "do it," as in…well, you know. I mean "do something other than 'it' that's fun."

We strongly recommend that you mark on a calendar a day and a time every week where each of you—you, your partner, and your sitter, if you have one—understands that this is your scheduled date. Don't have plans yet for those dates? No matter. You can always find something to do with that time. But if you don't schedule it and make it a weekly habit, it's much less likely to happen.

My interest in working with parents came from my own experiences during the early months after our first child was born. Our son was about three or four months old and I was working on Saturdays so that my husband, who worked weekdays, could stay with him. Since I made my own schedule, I worked around my husband's so that one of us could be home with our son. We hadn't been on a date since our first anniversary.

What? We hadn't been on a date since our first anniversary, when our son was three weeks old and we went out for 45 minutes before we had to come back. But other than that, we hadn't been out at all, just the two of us. We were definitely overdue.

Fortunately, my mom was visiting so we were able to have her watch our son that night. We went out just to get coffee and dessert but being able to talk—and we talked a lot about our son—made such a huge difference. I was able to remember why I loved spending time with my husband. We still had things in common and, most important, we both loved our son. It felt good to have that time together and to share stories to remind us why we wanted to have a child together. Stories like, "We had a wedding and everything. I almost forgot about that!"

Rick and I always encourage date night in our workshops, and I strongly encourage it during therapy sessions with new parents, even though we know how hard it can be to get out. It can be especially difficult if you don't have family or friends who can watch your baby and you need to hire someone. Plus, there's the additional cost of spending money on a date, which can be a problem given the expense of having a baby. So how can you find ways to make dating more feasible?

MAKE A LUNCH DATE

Kimberly and Alex were struggling to find time for each other. They both worked full time and the evenings were already filled up with chores; on weekends, they wanted to spend as much quality time as they could with their daughter. We talked about how they could fit in brief periods of time with each other—35 to 45 minutes several times a week add up over time.

They decided to meet once a week for lunch.

After several weeks, they reported an increased desire to spend more time together. They took off half days from work so that they didn't have to rush through a lunch, and they were even planning a mini getaway.

They also said the evenings that used to feel monotonous were more fun. After their daughter went to sleep, they seemed to have more time to spend either watching a show on Netflix or playing a game. They felt more connected and invested in each other. They were able to recognize ways that each of them was supporting the other.

The key thing here is to remember why you two love each other: something like, oh, yeah, you're fun and we laugh about stuff, and oh, yeah, we really have fun together.

For that first date, you don't have to go on a trip to France. Just go out together for an hour, then build up that trust.

ENDNOTES

23   Nancy Mohrbacher, *Breastfeeding Answers Made Simple: A Guide For Helping Mothers* (Amarillo: Hale Publishing, 2010), 489.

CHAPTER 4

The New Normal

Remember Steven and Ava, the couple you met in Chapter 2? Part of Ava's difficulty with finding balance as a parent was the enormous number of tasks she had to manage. It can become overwhelming for any new mother.

There are three questions that we ask participants in our workshops. Remember them from the introduction?

The first: "Are you taking care of yourself?" In other words, what do you need to do to make sure you're filling your cup—taking time for self-care—in order to get individual tasks done as well as to continue with ongoing tasks? This is a very important though difficult question for parents, especially moms, to answer. But remember, for you to be able to effectively take care of your family and enjoy doing it, you've first got to take care of you. We'll get into details in a bit.

The second: "What are you going to do to make sure that you're connecting with your partner to keep your relationship strong?" Many new parents will tell us that they just don't have it in them to complete one more "to-do" task. A lot of new moms who are working outside the home already feel guilty for not spending as much time with the baby as their stay-at-home friends do. Anyone who has to go to work, come home, make dinner, then get ready for the next day especially will roll their eyes at this question. Later we'll spend time breaking it all down.

The third: "How are you bonding with your baby?" This is usually easy for Mom to answer since most times bonding comes naturally. We ask the question to see if *both* partners are getting a chance to help with the baby, especially when we're dealing with a mom who likes to do it all, who has difficulty sharing tasks such as giving the baby baths, feeding the baby, or changing the baby's diapers.

If you spend all weekend cleaning, grocery shopping, and running errands in order to get ready for the work week, when, you might wonder, are you supposed to find time to take care of yourself and go on a date with your husband? Throwing all that into the mix, how are you supposed to get quality time with your baby?

Since we don't typically have the support we need, one of the best ways to balance all these undertakings is to create a schedule. And please know that when I say balance, I don't mean equal time, that is, always being able to devote one third of your time to work, another third to family, and still another third to self-care. Sometimes different parts of life demand more attention, which requires that you figure out what you need to meet your priorities.

I readily acknowledge that there are some parents (most) who don't want to create a schedule. It can feel contrived and chore-like to have to put date night on a calendar but honestly, it will make life easier. Especially until you get a better handle on all the things that need to be done and develop a more workable system for your family. Think of all the times you've said, "I've been meaning to…" Then you mention a task that easily could've been accomplished in the last few days, weeks, month, or even years but didn't get done because you didn't set aside time to accomplish it.

The same will happen with your self-care or date night if you don't block out the time.

AMY AND JOE'S STORY

Now that Amy had gone back to work, she struggled to balance everything. How was one human supposed to juggle a job, mothering, and partnering? Sure, she'd finally found childcare she was happy with. It was a bit of a drive, adding 15 minutes to her commute to work, but she was pleased with the child-to-care-worker ratio. She also was happy with the interactions she'd witnessed between the children and the workers. She was satisfied that her baby was being well taken care of. The constant negotiation with Joe about who was taking the baby to daycare and who was picking her up was still a hassle, though. And the bottle situation, which required her to pump each night for an hour, wasn't getting any better either.

The transition home with baby from daycare was chaotic and stressful. The baby continually cried and fussed in the car. She knew the baby was hungry because she was starving herself. That was only the beginning of the mad dash to accomplish everything she needed to do before she crashed for the night.

At home, Amy wolfed down crackers and cheese before she started dinner. Pouring herself a glass of wine, she considered the habit and figured she deserved a glass every now and then. She'd get the pump supplies cleaned and organized for the following day after she washed the dinner dishes. Lined up like little soldiers on the counter were the bottles that needed cleaning. She took a swig of wine. She still needed to remove the baby's dirty, pooped-on clothing from the diaper bag and load it with extra outfits and enough diapers for the next day.

This, of course, meant running a load of laundry and adding to the pile of unfolded clothes taking over the couch. The same couch upon which Joe now sat.

Joe called out, "What's for dinner?" She felt her skin crawl. With all the other tasks she needed to accomplish, she couldn't even think about cooking. Why couldn't he put something on the stove? Why did it have to be her? All she wanted to do was to cuddle and play with her sweet baby, who was beginning to giggle and coo more each day. Why did she have to miss all the good stuff?

But she knew that if she didn't start dinner, they wouldn't eat. Then it hit her. Not only did she have a million household chores to accomplish but she had work to catch up on, too, since she was having to leave the office 20 minutes early each day to pick up the baby on time. The last thing she needed was her employers thinking that she was slacking. These days she was continually arriving to the office late. The baby must have thrown up in the car on the way to daycare four times this week. Her manager had given her a dirty look because she'd missed three days in the last two months when the daycare thought that the baby had a fever.

Amy caught sight of her reflection in the microwave door. Her blouse wasn't buttoned correctly. She'd missed her regular salon appointment, the one she'd religiously kept every six to eight weeks. When was the last time she'd had her hair cut and colored? She poked at her flabby belly. Thanks to her cracker cravings, hell, her cravings for whatever she could put her hands on the minute she walked in the door, she'd never fit into her pre-pregnancy pants again.

Once she got the baby down for the night, all Amy wanted to do was lie down and go to sleep too. Unfortunately, the work wouldn't get done on its own. Amy glanced at Joe and felt a wave of envy surge in her chest. Sure, he'd taken on the dishes but now he got to chill and watch his favorite Netflix show.

Envy aside, part of her wanted to lie down next to him and cuddle. She missed their quiet time together. But another part of her knew that the second she lay down beside him, Joe would be putting the moves on her and she was so not ready for that. She couldn't remember the last time they had sex. Was it before she'd had the baby? Sex aside, Amy didn't even want to be touched. The thought horrified her. She didn't like how she looked or felt, and quite frankly, she was tired of being touched. All Amy really wanted was to fall face down on the bed and sleep for a solid week.

CREATE A SCHEDULE

It's important that you create a schedule. Mark on a calendar upcoming appointments, activities, and tasks such as household duties that need to get done and by whom. Be sure to schedule social support time and self-care time, as well as date night, a.k.a. time together without the baby.

It doesn't matter what you use, an old-fashioned paper calendar or a shared calendar system like Google, as long as it's something that works for your family and that you'll actually check.

For tasks that don't occur regularly, using a whiteboard or chalkboard or a smartphone app can be helpful. Create three columns: (1) Red – Do ASAP. (2) Yellow – Needs to happen soon. (3) Green – Put on the calendar to get done.

Many couples have told us that this has been extremely helpful since it limits the amount of nagging they feel compelled to engage in. They are clear on what they have agreed needs to be done, and when and if additional tasks become a concern or present themselves, those can be addressed in their regular check-ins, particularly when moms are looking for additional support.

STRESS

No one ever said life is easy. And adding a baby to the mix doesn't make it any easier; it adds enormous stress. In a report from the Pew Research Center, 40 percent of working moms said they always felt rushed, compared with 25 percent of working dads.[24] Stay-at-home moms, currently the minority in families with kids 17 or younger, were less rushed; however, 82 percent still said they experienced stress sometimes or frequently, compared with 86 percent of working moms and 74 percent of working dads.

It's important to recognize how stress can impact you. Are you able to recognize your stressors? Are you aware of them? What do you do to manage them?

The effect of stress on our bodies can be significant. In the short term, this depletion can lead to symptoms[25] such as:

- Fatigue

- Anxiety

- Depression

- Carbohydrate cravings

- Addictions

- Lack of focus

- Difficulty losing weight

- Difficulty sleeping

- Hormonal imbalance

Long-term health effects can be even more damaging—think hypertension or autoimmune disease. Like you've got time to worry about those things as well?

SELF-CARE 101

It's all about you, isn't it? The answer to that question is yes! Both parents are giving, giving, and giving some more. We have to take a little or we won't be able to give at all.

If you haven't already noticed that your roles as parents are constantly changing, you will soon enough. Babies and kids are great at keeping us on our toes! So a little flexibility and forgiving ourselves can go a long way. This is also true for our self-care routines.

It's so important to recognize that *self-care is not an indulgence*— it's as vital as making sure our kids are fed. I can't emphasize this enough. It can make all the difference in our ability to be patient, to use good judgment, to simply enjoy being a parent. We can't give our best when we don't feel our best.

Every person is different, every child has different needs, and every family has different values. Be secure in knowing that what you need to do for yourself and your family is the right thing.

Remember to talk with your partner about your need to be supported in order to make time for yourself. Ask how you, in turn, can support your partner so that they also get time for self-care.

WHAT WE MEAN BY SELF-CARE

As hard as it can be to give yourself permission to take time away from your children, it is so important because it ultimately will enable you to be more present with and for them. When we take care of ourselves, we tend to be more patient and more understanding.

Moreover, as a parent you want to be a good role model for your children. Start with modeling good self-care, and when they get older, they'll know what positive self-care looks like and they can grant themselves the permission to recharge their own batteries.

Nutrition. Be sure you're eating nutritional meals throughout the day, including proteins, complex carbs, and fats. Numerous books are available on the best nutrition while breastfeeding and beyond. Speak with your doctor if you have concerns about the quality of your diet.

Sleep. One study compared well-rested and sleep-deprived participants and the effect on their psyche. (I would've signed up for the well-rested group because I'm already familiar with the effects of sleep deprivation.) The researchers concluded that "when healthy participants were deprived of sleep and exposed to upsetting imag-es their brain activity had a similar reaction as depressed patients. And they had greater brain activity after viewing upsetting images than their well-rested counterparts, which is similar to the reac-tion that depressed patients have."[26] When we get limited sleep we then have limited time four our brain cells to replenish and our brain does not function as well, which can lead to a decrease in overall well-being and may increase the risk of developing a mood disorder like depression or anxiety.

Movement. Regular exercise has been proven to help reduce stress,[27] ward off anxiety[28] and feelings of depression,[29] boost self-esteem,[30] and improve sleep.[31] Fitness does not have to involve a rigorous, hour-long workout. Going outside for a walk, attending a yoga class, or putting on music and dancing around has been shown to do the trick. In other words, do something you enjoy that gets you moving and that you can fit into your crazy schedule.

Laughter. Research shows that laughing can reduce stress and ten-sion and decrease stress hormones while also boosting the immune system.[32] What can you do to ensure a good laugh?

- Watch funny movies.
- Read humorous books and materials.
- Be around friends who make you laugh.
- Find the humor in your children (e.g., your child's giggle or getting food all over their face).

Parenting Mentor(s). Parents who have older children, even by a few years, can give you the necessary encouragement. (More on this in Chapter 7.)

Beauty. Nourish your soul with aesthetics. Engage your senses to boost your mood.

- Sight: Add elements of beauty to the rooms you occupy most in your home. Decorate with things that you love, that stir wonder. Reduce clutter. Display artworks or nature scenes that appeal to you.

- Sound: Play music you enjoy, or listen to recordings of soothing nature sounds, e.g., rain falling or birds chirping. Get rid of sounds that displease you, e.g., beeping alarm clocks.

- Smell: Enhance your environment with your choice of a pleasant, subtle fragrance. Try lighting candles or adding potpourri to a room. Studies show that your sense of smell can influence your mood in a variety of ways. Peppermint can increase alertness, lavender is good for relaxation, etc. Don't be surprised if a scent you used to love no longer appeals to you. Pregnancy and postpartum are notorious for altering one's sense of smell.

A Spiritual Life. This is incredibly individual, yet important. Develop a prayer and/or meditation practice if only to acknowledge that, during the tough times, you'll get through it. Remember to slow down and trust yourself with where you are; don't succumb to the pressure you put on yourself by judging yourself against other parents. Do not push yourself to do more than what you or your body can handle. Be patient with yourself. And remember that you are a "good enough" mom just the way you are. All big changes take time to adjust to, so stay calm.

Part of having a healthy spiritual life, a positive attitude that will see you through the tough times, is developing a gratitude practice. We can be so hard on ourselves, on our partners, and on the people around us that we need to take time to acknowledge the good. Look around you.

Things to be grateful for:
- A patient partner
- Healthy children
- Happy children
- Flexibility in your schedule
- Supportive community that includes family and friends
- Safe neighborhood
- Access to healthcare
- Knowledge of where to find resources
- Ability to recognize when you need time for yourself
- Weekly date nights
- Weekly walks and lunch with office colleagues
- Monthly outings with girlfriends
- "Dance parties" with older children
- Binge-watching Netflix with spouse
- Friends who get what it's like to be a parent
- Friends without kids
- Parent groups
- Comfortable home
- Couch for cuddling with kids
- Couch for cuddling with partner
- Sunsets
- Sunrises
- Five o'clock p.m.
- Weekend getaways
- Family vacations
- Walking barefoot in the grass
- Baby's smiles
- Hugs
- Kisses
- Knowing glances

Saying No. One of the challenges with self-care is that it can feel like one more thing we need to do. Bringing home a baby already involves a million and one tasks, and we know that attending to our own needs can feel difficult to accomplish. But look at what your day looks like and ask yourself about each task, "Is this something that really needs to be done today [or at all]?"

Grace and Permission. You will never be able to do it all. And so, you need to let go of that impossible standard. You need help. You need support. Sometimes you just need a break. And some days you'll be better at self-help than others. That's OK. Remember, your children, your partner, and your friends don't need you to be perfect. They need you to be real.

MIKE'S STORY

Mike was a brand-new father and really struggling to find his role as a dad. It seemed that his wife was always taking care of the baby; she spent so much time feeding their son, all he felt he got to do was change diapers. Plus, when he did try to interact with the baby, the baby didn't seem to respond much. Mike shared that even though he loved his son, he honestly thought babies were boring.

We discussed ways that Mike could incorporate time with the baby into things he enjoyed, like working out. Mike's routine was to hit the gym daily for an hour or so but realistically that wasn't an option at this time, at least not on a daily basis. He figured out how he could work out while spending time with his son—he would take his son for a long walk to the neighborhood park where he would do some kind of quick, high-intensity interval training. He soon realized that there were plenty of things he could do with his son, and he started incorporating the baby into his day and the chores he did around the house. It wasn't long before he started getting smiles and giggling responses from his son, and it made everything that much more enjoyable.

WHY SELF-CARE WORKS

Research consistently shows that parents must balance their needs with those of their children for the best health outcomes.[33] It sounds noble to sacrifice one's self for the sake of one's children but no one survives self-emollition.

It's not all or nothing. If each of you puts time on the calendar for a few self-care practices, you're that much closer to creating balance for everyone involved.

One of the difficulties with getting self-care time, especially with a newborn, is that we often can't think of exactly what we want to do when the time presents itself. So I encourage parents to make a list of things they would like to do or would enjoy doing once the opportunity arises. Think of things you can do if you have 5 minutes, 15 minutes, 30 minutes, or more.

- Identify five things Dad needs per week to support his self-care (e.g., playing basketball with friends, going to the gym, reading a book, watching a favorite show) and his health (e.g., a nutritious lunch, exercise, at least six hours of sleep per night).

- Identify five things Mom needs per week to support her self-care (e.g., taking a walk with a friend, going to the gym, reading a book, watching a favorite show) and her health (e.g., a nutritious lunch, exercise, at least six hours of sleep per night).

- Identify five things Mom and Dad need together to maintain the health of their relationship (e.g., daily check-ins, nightly walks, weekly dates, quarterly nights away, yearly getaways).

This is where you're able to incorporate the three questions that we mentioned in the introduction. So for everything you have to do, what are the items you are adding to your calendar to answer: (1) What are you going to do to take care of yourself? (2) What are you going to do to take care of your relationship? (3) What are you doing to bond with your child?

RICK'S TAKE

We were not smart enough in our son's first year to ask ourselves the three questions that Catherine has outlined here. But through dumb luck, we fell into practices that answered these questions. One of the things we stumbled upon was bath time.

In our son's first year, I was the one who gave him a bath. I have no idea how that happened but it was the best part of my day. I looked forward to having time with him when we could just hang out and be together without distraction. It also was the time of day when Catherine knew that she could take 10 to 20 minutes for herself.

So with little real thought, I was able to answer what I was doing to bond with the baby and what I was doing to take care of my partner.

ENDNOTES

24   "The Decline of Marriage And Rise of New Families," Pew Research Center report, accessed June 5, 2020, https://www.pewsocialtrends.org/2010/11/18/the-decline-of-marriage-and-rise-of-new-families/.

25   Ann Pietrangelo et al., "The Effects of Stress on Your Body," accessed June 5, 2020, https://www.healthline.com/health/stress/effects-on-body#1.

26   Els van der Helm et al., "Overnight Therapy? The Role of Sleep in Emotional Brain Processing," *The Psychological Bulletin* 135, no. 5, (2009): 731–748, https://doi.org/10.1037/a0016570.

27   "Exercising to relax," Harvard Health Publishing, last modified July 13, 2018, accessed June 5, 2020, https://www.health.harvard.edu/staying-healthy/exercising-to-relax.

28   Elizabeth Anderson et al., "Effects of Exercise and Physical Activity on Anxiety," *Frontiers in Psychiatry* (2013), https://doi.org/10.3389/fpsyt.2013.00027

29   Gary Cooney et al., "Exercise for Depression," *JAMA* 311, no. 23 (June 2014), https://doi.org/10.1001/jama.2014.4930.

30   Seyed Hojjat Zamani Sani et al., "Physical Activity and Self-Esteem: Testing Direct and Indirect Relationships Associated with Psychological and Physical Mechanisms," *Neuropsychiatric Disease and Treatment* (2016), https://doi.org/10.2147/NDT.S116811.

31   Jessica R. Alley, "Effects of Resistance Exercise Timing on Sleep Architecture and Nocturnal Blood Pressure," *The Journal of Strength and Conditioning Research* 29, no. 5 (2015): 1378-1385, https://doi.org/10.1519/JSC.0000000000000750.

32   Lawrence Robinson et al., "Laughter is the Best Medicine," Help Guide, last modified November 2019, accessed June 8, 2020, https://www.helpguide.org/articles/mental-health/laughter-is-the-best-medicine.htm.

33   Martha Okafor et al., "Improving Health Outcomes of Children through Effective Parenting: Model and Methods," *International Journal of Environmental Research and Public Health* 11, no. 1 (December 2013): 296-311, https://doi.org/10.3390/ijerph110100296.

CHAPTER 5

It's a Baby, Not a Basketball: Don't Pass It

The changes you experience when baby comes home are imme-diate and drastic. Often, you try to keep doing what you've always done while fitting this new priority into your schedule. The problem is that time is limited and this drastically affects your communication with each other.

TIM AND JEANNIE'S STORY

Tim had to deal with Jeannie feeling overwhelmed early on when he arrived home from work. She was working, too, but was self-employed. During her work hours, the baby would stay with her mother and it wasn't until Tim got home that she'd tell him she hadn't gone to pick up the baby. She was busy handling some work-related activity, though it seemed like she was just talking on the phone. Tim would have to wait to find out if he was going to be sent out to pick up the baby, even though he could've done it on the way home.

TIM'S PERSPECTIVE

I don't know why it is so hard for Jeannie to send me a text to pick up the baby on my way home from work. It could save a lot of wasted time and we could actually spend more time together as a family.

JEANNIE'S PERSPECTIVE

One of these days, I'm going to get done with work on time and surprise Tim and be home with the baby so we can make dinner together or go out. I always get caught up in what I'm doing. I wish he'd send me a text that he's on his way so I can give him a heads-up to get the baby.

Someone has to take the lead and communicate. That way, both Tim's and Jeannie's expectations are more likely to be met.

It's not uncommon to feel like you and your partner hardly ever see each other, especially considering that one or both of you have to go to work. If you've been at home with the baby all day, you might be desperate for a break by the time your partner comes home. When you return from work, your partner might need to dash off to a meeting. Sometimes it can feel like the two of you are just passing the baby back and forth. While it's nice that you have each other to rely on to care for the baby (it's a heck of a lot cheaper than hiring a babysitter), you probably feel like you rarely see each other.

If you rarely see each other, that means baby rarely sees you together. So don't always take turns. Be sure that there's time for the family unit, not just for baby. Make dinner time sacred, even if your little one isn't eating table food yet. Or if you're really pressed for time, read a book or sing a song together.

One of the things we often hear is that one partner feels like they are doing everything. And typically it's the mom who shares that she is feeling this way. There's the frustration that she is always having to ask for help. That it isn't obvious to her partner what needs to be done. That her partner doesn't do the things she asked him to do just yesterday. Moms report feeling like they carry the Mental Load of Parenting.[34]

Even when a partner does help, it can feel like a lot of managing. Then add the frustration that the couple still is not doing things together and is missing spending time as a family unit.

Here are questions to ask yourselves to explore ways to spend more time together while also getting things done:

- How can we manage all our chores/activities together?
- How can we incorporate the baby in the things we have to do together?

The prospect of going out into the world was daunting. I could barely cope with getting the baby cleaned, dressed and fed in the privacy of my own home. How could I handle breast feeding, or a diaper blow out in public?

I remember dreading the day my husband went back to work because he was the one who had prior experience with babies. I surely didn't. I had babysat a few kids but the only time I ever had to change a diaper my mom had come over and rescued me from the task.

I wasn't sure how my sweet little boy and I were going to get through the days at home all by ourselves. I also knew that I couldn't just be home all day, every day. I needed people to talk to and socialize with. I was used to being on the go and having a lot of things to do each day.

I Can Do This! Wait, No I Can't

I had a good heart-to-heart with myself about what I felt I needed during this time. I needed to feel competent as a mom and not feel isolated. I knew that meant I was going to have to get out of the house because all my friends were working and couldn't come hang out with me all day.

I was worried about changing diapers in public, worried that my baby would cry and I wouldn't be able to console him. What about breastfeeding? I was struggling enough at home, how was I going to breastfeed in public?

That's when I decided to compile a list of what I considered baby-friendly places. Isn't it amazing that they are so hard to find? Where is their identifying sign? Restaurants are vegan friendly, gluten-free friendly, and just plain friendly, except to mothers who have a newborn. I want a sign out in front showing a mom holding a baby.

I made my list of baby-friendly places where I imagined other people would not be bothered if I changed a diaper or if my baby cried or needed to be fed.

I looked into where groups for moms met, and fortunately one was offered through the hospital where I had delivered my son. So I put that on my list. Then there was the place where I had been practicing prenatal yoga. They also offered postpartum classes where you could bring your baby with you. Perfect!

Those could be my starting places while I grew in competency. Eventually, I would be able to handle going shopping or taking my son to a restaurant. I figured I could get used to caring for him outside the comfort of my home and see how I handled the stressful situations of his crying or having a diaper blowout.

Plus, I quickly realized that I was able to pick up a lot of tips on how to do things easier by watching other moms interact and care for their babies.

This is just one of the many reasons that I decided to start a new parent meetup group. I wasn't the only one benefiting from the support and encouragement. I've had mom after mom tell me that hearing another mom share her struggle or success helped to give her confidence to try something else—to realize that there isn't just one way to do something.

You Can Still Do What You Love
One of the concerns we hear from parents is that their life is going to be over once the baby comes. They'll stop doing the things they enjoy.

And so, part of taking baby steps is to start incorporating the baby into some of the things you do. We've had couples who have shared that they go camping but their camping involves backpacking five miles to set up camp beside a backcountry lake. You're probably not doing that with an infant. (Maybe some people do. I'm sure we will get an e-mail from someone who has rappelled down a mountain with their baby, who of course spit up on their shoulder.)

For the most part, the people we've talked to feel like they have to give it all up, saying, "We don't know when we'll ever get to go camping again."

You need to adapt your activities to the new reality. So the five-mile hike backpacking to a campsite is now maybe car camping. But this is not forever. As your baby grows and your skills increase, that car camping can become a short hike to a campsite and then before you know it, a five-mile hike backpacking as a family unit to the campsite.

Part of the problem is that we often don't know what we don't know—especially if this is our first baby. It's pretty difficult to prepare for something if we don't know that's part of the deal. And even if we are super prepared, we'll still have those days where we're exhausted and at our wit's end no matter how helpful our partners are.

Will you get frustrated and angry with your partner? Will you find yourself keeping score about who's doing what and how much they're doing? Will the things you used to take for granted seem like an out-of-reach luxury?

Yes to all those things.

But (and it's a big but) there are ways you can make sure that your life with your partner does not end after baby comes home. Fair warning: you'll have to work at it.

Does it take more effort to spend time with your partner? Will you have to make a conscious effort to connect with each other, possibly even scheduling couples time on the calendar? Will there be times that you'd rather be sleeping than having a "date?"

Yes to all of those!

It is so important to make sure that you spend time together. Committing to checking in with each other helps you in ways that aren't immediately apparent. It helps you to stay connected to each other. It helps you to listen to each other. It helps you to explain what you feel in a level-headed way. It helps you to reprioritize when things aren't working. It helps you to recharge your emotional batteries. And it helps you to be better parents because you feel heard, understood, and supported.

ACKNOWLEDGE UNEXPECTED LOSS

One of the things I want to make clear is that it is okay to feel in parenthood a sense of loss. This is something that is often not talked about. In fact, I've counseled couples who describe their sadness, anger, frustration, etc., and don't realize why until we start exploring how they are feeling. They've been told to expect feeling excited for this amazing time in their lives, this addition to their family. "It's gonna be awesome! Enjoy every minute!"

We talk about getting ready for all the newness—the birth, the baby's first steps, the baby's first words—but soon Mom and Dad are in a kind of endless loop where everything seems to be the same day after day. They start to notice all the things they don't get to do anymore or realize the difficulty in doing the things that used to be so much simpler. The spontaneity is gone. And even though they love their child so much—and believe me, I know that they do—the guilt they experience for feeling like they're missing out and the resentment they harbor for not being able to catch up with their friends during happy hour are very real.

So how do you combat those feelings of loss?

- **Identify what you're feeling.** Becoming aware of and naming our emotions can help us to express our feelings. This helps us to move past our difficult feelings more easily.

- **Feel the feeling.** No matter if we are feeling sadness, anger, or even happiness, it is important to be aware of whatever feeling it is so that we can help identify what we may need for ourselves in this situation.

- **Acknowledge that this is part of becoming a parent.** You are not alone in how you are feeling.

- **Remember that you will not always feel this way.** Everything changes, and with time so will this.

ENDNOTES

34   Jessica Grose, "A Modest Proposal for Equalizing the Mental Load," the *New York Times*, June 11, 2019, accessed June 8, 2020, https://www.nytimes.com/2019/06/11/parenting/mental-load.html.

CHAPTER 6

When You Haven't Showered in Three Days

In those early days of bringing home a baby, everything slows down but there also seems to be so much more work to do. Often, parents will share that they feel like they can't do anything the way they used to. Let's talk about tasks and how you might accomplish them in unique ways.

CLAIRE AND DAVID'S STORY

Claire and David shared how they seemed to spend so much time taking care of their new baby. It felt like all they managed to get done was nursing and changing diapers and their baby would sleep only if he was being held by one of them. They had begun to wonder why they had purchased a crib because the baby had never been in it for more than a few minutes.

They were struggling to figure out how they were supposed to get everything done. They described a tag team of sorts to accomplish tasks: Claire would start on the dishes while David held the baby while the baby slept, but then the baby would wake up and need to nurse so David would pass the baby off to her. David would then start to do some laundry but partway through that task, Claire would finish nursing and want to get up and move around so David would sit down to hold the baby again while the baby slept. They were playing a new version of hot potato! It felt like an endless cycle. There were half-done chores all around the house and they both felt tired and unproductive, but the plus side was that their baby was well-fed, happy, and dressed better than they were.

Those early days can feel like scenes from the movie *Groundhog Day*. How can you start to figure out how to incorporate the baby into the things you do?

Claire and David soon learned that they would have more time to spend together when they did some of their chores with the baby. David started "wearing" his son in a carrier while he was vacuuming, and Claire would put the baby in a bouncy seat while she was folding clothes or making dinner. The baby being close by and listening to her voice seemed to buy Claire some time.

Gradually, you can move babies farther away from you and they'll still feel safe and secure. You may be able to keep them comfortable with your being out of their line of sight by playing peekaboo as you move around.

WHY CAN HE GET THINGS DONE, BUT I CAN'T?

We've had many moms say they feel frustrated that their partners seem to get things done but they can't. I experienced this with my husband. He could get a lot done with our kids when they were babies, but I didn't seem to be able to accomplish anything past nursing and feeding, which, don't get me wrong, is a lot!

RICK'S TAKE

I believe that I was more comfortable in the beginning with our son fussing and crying. I did not drop everything just because he cried. I would certainly check on him and make sure that he was safe, clean, and fed. But I would not stop to hold our son if I was cleaning something or loading the dishwasher. I knew that taking the 30 seconds to finish what I was doing was not going be harmful to our son. I also knew that seeing to him without the distraction of worrying about what I had not completed meant I was more present when I did attend to him.

I also tried to find ways to incorporate our son into whatever chore I was doing. For example, I would bring him into the kitchen and place him somewhere where he could see me. I would then talk to him about the dishes I was cleaning and putting away. Doing this was a way to complete the task and at the same time bond with our son.

MAKE A DAILY TASK LIST

Often, when someone asks what you need help with, in that moment it can seem like everything's under control, so you say, "Nothing. I'm fine." That's very brave of you but don't! Instead, you can hand them a list and ask them to choose something from it. You have so much going on and so many people want to help or have offered to help, why not let them? That way, you have one less decision to make and they don't feel forced to do something they don't want to do.

It's time to make a daily task list. I know that you're thinking how fun this is going to be—this is why you bought the book!

The good news is that it's already done for you—*poof!* Just look below. (Later we will talk about how to accomplish tasks if you don't have much help.)

Daily Task List

- Making grocery list: What are your staple items? Can you double recipes and eat leftovers? What brands do you use?
  - Milk
  - Vegetables
  - Fruits
  - Snacks (Consider things that are easy to grab while your nursing but are also nutritious)
  - Breakfast
  - Lunch
  - Dinner
- Grocery shopping
- Buying diapers
- Paying bills: water, electric, car, house/mortgage/rent, child-care, etc.
- Washing baby's things: toys, reusable diapers, bottles
- Washing pumping equipment
- Cleaning the kitchen
- Wiping down counters
- Preparing meals
- Cooking
- Washing dishes
- Cleaning out dishwasher
- Cleaning bedrooms
- Changing linens
- Washing clothes, linens, towels

- Folding laundry
- Cleaning bathroom(s): toilet, shower, sink, floor
- Vacuuming
- Sweeping
- Dusting
- Car care: washing, filling up with gas, changing oil, performing other maintenance
- Lawn care: mowing (how frequently), fertilizing, aerating, watering
- Plant care: fertilizing, pruning, watering
- Gardening: fertilizing, planting seeds, picking vegetables and fruit
- Raking leaves
- Running errands
- Paying bills
- Taking care of pets: feeding, washing, walking the dog

Often, people will ask you what they can do for you. This is when you can hand them your list of things that you're comfortable having people do for you.

One of my clients put together a spreadsheet before the birth of her first child. At her baby shower, she had people sign up for different tasks like cleaning the bathroom or mowing the lawn or bringing meals and they actually loved it. She said they liked being able to know what they could do to help out and to sign up for the things they could do without feeling pressured.

Go to HappyWithBaby.com to download your customizable spreadsheet.

You Will Need Help...But From Whom?

Many websites can help you throughout the difficult moments of parenting. Look for articles about the developmental stages of your baby and about common illnesses or symptoms, and also look for tips and support. Of course, I'm going to recommend my own website: HappyWithBaby.com. *Remember, be selective about what you read; if it only serves to make you doubt yourself, close it down!*

At first, you'll want to tackle a few of the chores on your daily task list. You may be able to slip one or two of them into your day, particularly as the baby grows older. Do not, however, try to take them all on. All that you could do before you had a child is now no longer realistic, or advisable.

Slow down and trust yourself with where you are. Don't push yourself to do more than what you can do, physically or emotionally. You just had a baby and the Pilates class you used to do prior to becoming pregnant and the hike your best friend is doing with her partner and baby may not be something you can take on at this point and that is perfectly ok. You will get back to your ability "to move mountains," but when you go slower getting there, you learn and accomplish a great deal more and cope a lot better.

And it doesn't matter what you hear that other parents are doing. You aren't getting the full story. Remember, your situation is unique. You can't care what the rest of the world is doing. Listen to your own heart!

Be patient with yourself about what you want to do and what you need to do. For those necessary tasks you dislike, ask yourself the following questions:

- Can I change them? Can I get help? Will my partner shoulder some of the tasks?

- If I can't change them now, can I make a plan to eventually take them off my list of things I have to do myself? Identify long-term goals, e.g., how long you will be nursing through the night. Three more weeks? Six more months? Mark a date on the calendar. If the date comes and you are not ready or the date feels too overwhelming, you can always adjust it.

- Can I find ways to make them more enjoyable? Focus on tasks you like, for example, bathing your baby or watching your baby sleep. Allow those to be present when you are doing tasks you find unpleasant. Also, consider other ways you might make an unpleasant task more enjoyable, e.g., lighting aromatic candles, opening windows and letting in fresh air, or listening to music, a podcast, or an audiobook.

- Can I prioritize them?

Now that you've identified the few tasks that you must do or are willing to do, what about the rest? This is where you learn to delegate. Delegating isn't just something you do at the office; it's something you must learn to do in life.

The list of tasks that come with the arrival of your baby seems to increase exponentially and as they get older the list does not necessarily decrease. Trying to do it all on your own often leads you to fail or to feel so overwhelmed that you break down. It often starts with your partner trying to help you out but they don't do things quite the way you would so you take over. They give up trying because they are tired of hearing you complain that they don't fold the shirts right or that they don't load the dishwasher properly or that they forgot to dust the entertainment center.

And honestly, that may be true, but the fact is, they will do things differently. You need their help. Plus, they need to help. They need to feel like they are useful.

It's likely that you helped someone when they had a baby. It's also likely that you will be asked in the future to help. So why not get yourself a little help now?

Ask yourself:

- Who can help?
- Whom have I helped with their baby?
- Can I trade services with someone?
- Can I divide up tasks with my partner based on what each likes doing better?
- What can I stop doing for now?

Right now, you don't need to solve every concern that you've identified. And you don't need to do it all on your own. We're about to indicate sources of support.

Are there people in your circle who will be more than happy to help and you don't even have to ask them? They'll just jump in and start doing stuff. Then there are people who won't offer to do anything and won't be helpful at all.

HERE'S A SURPRISE TWIST

Two wonderful people in my life are a good example of the complexity of getting help.

My mother will do anything and everything and you don't even have to ask but you might not necessarily like what she does. My mother-in-law will do absolutely nothing until you ask her. (They're both completely fine that I put this in the book, I hope.)

The reason that my mother-in-law wanted me to ask her each and every time for help with the baby—which was a bit frustrating, to say the least—was that (I found out later) she didn't want to step on my toes. I'm thinking, just step on my toes and do something, like my mother does! Except, every time my mother did something, I thought, "Why did she do it that way?" She just wanted to show me a way she thought was better. Do you see the problem? I didn't take into consideration where each of them was coming from.

PRETEND THEY MEAN WELL BECAUSE THEY PROBABLY DO
I recently had a client who was super frustrated because her mother-in-law would basically tell her how to do things by saying how she raised her kids. My client felt belittled. Her husband talked to his mother about it, and she was like, "Oh no, I was just trying to relate to her." She wasn't judging how her daughter-in-law was parenting. She was trying to relate to her by sharing from her own experience.

If you're feeling like someone in your life is critiquing you and analyzing everything you do and how you're not doing it right, pause, then take a deep breath because often it's coming from a place of support. Their perspective may be that they want things to be easier for you or that they want to be helpful and share something they used to do.

Now there are those who might interpret the advice as being really great, while others might interpret it as really stressful. It often depends on how you're receiving it. It can cause stress. It can cause anxiety. It can cause frustration. It can cause you to doubt yourself.

So it is important that you're able to talk to family or friends and let them know how you feel and what you need. Explain that you appreciate their suggestions but that you're trying to figure things out on your own as new parents. You'll take their suggestions into consideration but for now you're going to do things your way and see how that works. As you find your way as new parents and figure out your roles, you'll look into other ideas and you'll try different things. You acknowledge their ideas, but you have a plan, and being inundated with suggestions at this time is not helpful. You will be sure to ask when you need some advice.

Sometimes we accept people's help but we're not specific and straightforward with them about the kind of help we need because in the beginning we might not even be sure what that looks like.

Once you figure out what support you need, it is important to ask and be direct about it. People won't always do what you ask but if you don't ask, they most likely won't do what you want. They don't always know what isn't helpful either. So it's important to be specific and direct about the ways you need support.

Now we definitely know that is not always easy. It's important that if something someone is saying is bothering you, you are able to let them know how you feel. If it is too difficult to bring the situation up to someone like your mother-in-law, it is good to get your partner to help you navigate those difficult conversations.

CHAPTER 7

I'm Batmom, Not Supermom

Where do you turn for help? Because you *will* need support. Please, don't be a Supermom. We mentioned this before and we hear it from a lot of new parents, especially moms who feel like asking for help is somehow a weakness: "I'm weak. I should be able to do this. I see other moms on Instagram doing everything. I'm struggling to even get a shower and they're out taking pictures at the local zoo with their babies. I'm clearly failing at this motherhood thing. If I ask for help, everyone is going to know that I'm not enjoying every minute and that I'm not a good-enough mom. Especially when there are all those Supermoms out there. They probably even have a Fortress of Solitude. What do I have?"

Well, sweet momma, it's time you realize that you're Batmom. This isn't about being from another planet and born with invincible powers. Motherhood is about having tools in your toolbelt, having a great sidekick, and looking good in tights. Batmom is just as cool as Supermom (and some—Rick and my kids—would say it's even cooler) because she has to work at it. She always has a plan to try and figure out how to make things better and work smoother.

If you're feeling like you're not Supermom, you are definitely not alone, but it's time to call on your support system, a.k.a. side-kicks. Like Robin, who is always willing to help out in any way and has your back. Or like Commissioner Gordon, who is wise and can see what's not working and offer ideas for a different plan. Then there is Lucius Fox, who is super creative and artistic and can make great outfits. Or Alfred, Batman's butler—yeah, yeah, we know that most of us can't afford a butler, but what about saying yes when someone offers you a hand? Listen for it, they are offering. Think about who these people are in your life. Maybe they're a support group. And just maybe going to the support group or talking with other moms, you'll realize that you're not alone in your feelings of inadequacy and you can stop thinking that you have to try and aspire to be Supermom.

Marla and Marcus' Story

After a particularly stressful night of the baby waking every 45 minutes—or maybe it was stressful because it felt like the mil-lionth night in a row the baby woke every 45 minutes to eat or have her diaper changed—Marla seriously wondered if she'd ever sleep again. She was exhausted and frustrated. She didn't know how the hell she and Marcus had gotten themselves into this situation. It had been two months and she had only one more month left of maternity leave. Things didn't seem to be getting that much easier.

She was feeling frantic at the thought of going back to work. How could she do that when she was barely making it through the day now? And the thing was, part of her was looking forward to going back to work because at least then she'd be able to talk to adults and discuss things other than poop and spit up.

Plus, her coworkers might even notice the great job she was do-ing and compliment her. *Oh gawd!* She hoped she'd be able to function and be the outstanding employee she used to be.

Then there was the huge part of her—the guilty part—that didn't want to go back to work. She wanted to be the one to take care of her baby; she thought that each and every time she looked at her sweet, adorable sleeping baby. She wanted to be the one to experience all the firsts: the first mouthful of solid food, the first step, the first word, the first everything. *What kind of mother goes to all the trouble of having a baby and then runs off to work?* Marcus would be pissed at her if she changed her mind. They'd discussed the work situation endlessly prior to giving birth and she had told him that she would go back to her job and bring in a paycheck. They already had plans for how they'd spend the money.

But who the hell was she going to trust with this baby? They had checked out daycares and interviewed nannies but she didn't even trust Marcus to take care of their baby, not the way she did anyway. How was she going to trust a total stranger with her only child?

These thoughts and worries brought her to tears. There were more tears when she considered even more what-ifs: What if the house caught on fire while she was out of the house? What if there was an emergency and she wasn't there to take care of the baby? What if the baby was crying and she wasn't around to soothe her? What if a daycare worker or nanny didn't take care of the baby the way she would?

When Marcus got home, he found her crying on the couch. He sat down next to her and asked her what was wrong. She blubbered about not wanting to leave the baby.

He said they'd figure something out but Marla felt like he didn't mean it. She could tell by his tone.

"Do you think this is easy for me?" she asked. "Do you think I enjoy staying home while you go off to work every day and have lunch with your buddies? Do you know how hard it is to do the same thing day in and day out without so much as a thank you?"

She felt angry just looking at his blank face. "This is so hard. I love our baby so much that I can't even imagine anyone else taking care of her. I don't know what I'd do if something happened to her. But I also miss my old life and feeling competent at my job." She burst out into fresh tears.

Marcus returned the fire. Did she understand how hard it was for him too? But Marla couldn't hear him, couldn't sympathize with him, because clearly he had things easier.

She felt like Marcus wasn't being helpful and, worse, every time she'd ask him for help, he'd snap at her. She couldn't remember him ever being so abrasive and harsh toward her.

The baby started to cry. Marcus got up off the couch. After several moments he brought the baby into the living room, wearing one sock and with drool trickling down her chin. Marcus didn't seem to notice any of this. The baby would catch her death of cold and get that horrible rash thing on her face.

Marla felt horrible for resenting Marcus. She felt horrible for wanting and then not wanting to go back to work. She felt horrible that she hadn't slept in ages or felt like a human being for months.

Marla needed some support; she knew this. She needed a community to help validate all these feelings she was having. She needed to talk to someone. She needed someone to tell her that things were going to be OK. She needed someone to tell her that it would get easier. She needed someone to tell her that she was doing a good job and that mothering was hard.

MY OWN NEED FOR EMOTIONAL SUPPORT
When our first child was about four months old, I returned to my private practice as a Licensed Marriage and Family Therapist. My husband and I had altered our schedules so that when he was at work during the day I was at home with our son and vice versa. That meant I would go to work for a few hours in the evenings after

he got home and on Saturdays so that he could stay with our son.

One fateful Saturday morning, I was getting ready for work and we got into a terrific fight. To this day, I can't remember what the fight was about, I only know it had left me in tears as I drove to work.

I felt like shit. How the hell was I supposed to help other couples in my private practice when I couldn't even figure out how to help us? We'd been bickering more and more. On top of it all, everything Rick did seemed to drive me crazy.

There was the constant worry and guilt about going back to work or not going back to work, about what was best for our son and what was best for us as a unit. I knew I had it easy on many levels in that, because of the nature of my work, I could adjust my schedule. I also had a husband willing and able to do the same. And yet my days were filled with worry: Worry about going to work when I was at home with the baby, then worry about him when I was at work. I would hear endless news stories about terrible things happening to babies and small children, which only served to exponentially increase my anxiety.

What kind of mother was I if I wasn't going to be taking care of my own child?

Like Marla, I needed help. I needed support. I needed an expert's perspective. That's when I decided to call my girlfriend because she had kids who were older. She'd been at this game for five years or so. She'd know what to do. It also didn't hurt that she was a therapist too.

Through my tears, I explained to her what was going on: The guilt, the nonstop bickering with Rick. As all good friends and therapists do, she listened and validated my feelings and my experience. Then she asked me a single question: "When was the last time you and Rick were on a date?"

PARENTING MENTOR

Which brings us to the next very related topic. It's important to get help with the day-to-day tasks but often it's almost more important to have someone at the ready for emotional support, someone other than your partner or a parent, someone who's been in your shoes before.

This is the person you can bounce ideas off of. The person who can reassure you when you're feeling lonely or constantly questioning your role as a new parent. Having a support system is crucial, especially if you don't have family nearby.

It's also important that this trusted confidant be someone who's nonjudgmental, compassionate, and caring. (Being able to receive loving feedback is more comforting than you might imagine.) Someone who's been there but isn't in the thick of it. Someone you can model, not compare yourself with.

I lapped up my friend's advice because I knew she'd been there before. I also knew she wasn't judging me in that very moment the way I was judging myself.

GROUP SUPPORT

I've had several clients tell me that until they started going to a moms group, they didn't realize they weren't the only ones struggling. The other mothers also had issues with breastfeeding, trying to get their baby to sleep, or just feeling isolated and alone during the day.

How empowering it was to realize that they were all in the same "Batboat" with other moms. They weren't all defective mothers. They weren't enjoying every single moment because it's impossible to enjoy every single moment, and there were other moms who were having that same experience.

How helpful it was to be around all the sidekicks and to learn from them and feel their support. I thought, "I may not be a Supermom, I'm much better. I'm Batmom!"

Part II:
Taking Care of Your Relationship

CHAPTER 8

Prioritizing Your Relationship

This is a strange baby book, isn't it? It's focused on your relationship with your significant other. You keep expecting advice on bottles, burping, and baby food.

The world has suddenly become all about your baby. You're like the invisible couple. Even when a book may be about the two of you, in your mind, it's still about the baby. Let's make sure we get that straightened out right now.

I may get a lot of pushback on this but it's important that you understand why it's so vital to strengthen your relationship when a new baby has entered the picture. After all, babies have a *lot* of needs.

You've worked out which responsibilities each of you as a couple handles, but now you have a new member of the family who needs you to handle everything. This little one has no idea how to divide up responsibilities, and often you end up doing things for the baby that no one negotiated and it's left to whoever feels like doing it.

That's why you need to prioritize your relationship so that you can figure this stuff out together. The challenge is that when baby is here, it seems impossible to make time to do this. You are scrambling to figure out how to take care of this tiny human. The relationship can wait. But no, it can't.

Seven Reasons Why You Should Prioritize Your Relationship

1. I've yet to meet a true Supermom or Superdad. I have met some who've tried to be super. Every one of them has experienced some very real repercussions from trying to do it all. You're supposed to be doing this together. If you were hanging artwork, you'd ask for help: "Honey, is this straight?" (Unless you like artwork hung crookedly.) None of us can do it all without help.

2. Though this might be the last thing on your mind right now, kids eventually do move out. When your child walks out the door to go to college, you don't want to look at the other occupant of your home and wonder, "Who is this person?" and frantically dial 911. Even before that, your child likely will have a sleepover at a family member's or a friend's house, and it's helpful to remember the reason you chose this person to have a child with. They're pretty fun and you fell in love with them. We're talking about the person who chose to commit to you for life.[35] You made and chose to have a baby with this person so it's important that you don't forget their needs.

3. Kids learn by watching what we do, not hearing what we say (though they do seem to catch on to some things we may wish they didn't). The best way to teach children to consider others, work through problems, and understand what love and healthy relationships look like is by showing them. (Which is the same reason you don't take your children golfing until they're much older.)

4. Speaking of kids learning by what we do, a lot of us have never had a healthy marriage or partnership modeled for us. That

is why we need to take time now to learn how to nurture the relationship.

5. You're so many things besides just "mother" or "father" or "breadwinner" or "runner of households and all things domestic." Your needs, desires, aspirations, and well-being matter too. That includes companionship, intimacy, and yes, even sex and pleasure. Even if those feel less urgent right now to one of you.

6. When Mom isn't OK, it's harder for everyone else to be OK. If a mom doesn't feel supported and understood, her risk for postpartum depression and other mood and anxiety disorders increases. Science suggests that mom's mental health affects baby's development.[36] And it increases the risk for postpartum depression in dads as well. This (among so many other reasons) is why it's so important for partners to understand how to support and prioritize each other.

7. Long-term marital discord affects a child's mental health as the child grows older. Studies show links between frequent or aggressive arguments between parents and their children's development of unhealthy perfectionism, anxiety, social dysfunction, mood problems, and trauma, not to mention impaired problem-solving and struggling academically in school.[37]

Take time to reread this list and commit it to memory. It is that important to prioritize your partner!

JENNIFER AND MATT'S STORY

New parents to a baby girl, Jennifer and Matt came to a recent workshop that Rick and I were conducting.

JENNIFER'S PERSPECTIVE

What is wrong with me? Why is this so freaking hard? I clearly wasn't meant to be a mom. I can't seem to get anything accomplished. I spend all day trying to breastfeed and it's a nightmare. The pain hasn't seemed to go away even though I've been breathing deeply all day long. They say I'm not doing it right but I've talked to all the specialists. My clothes—who am I kidding, my pajamas, which I've been wearing for an entire week—are stained with spit up and God only knows what else. I cringe when Matt tries to sneak in for a kiss; I don't want him to touch me like this. I just want to take a long, hot shower and come out looking like the moms I see on Instagram. But I'm honestly too exhausted to do anything and it's only 9:00 a.m. Matt is already showered, dressed, and off to work. He seems to have it so easy. Plus, he gets praise from everyone for what a wonderful dad he is.

It wasn't supposed to be like this. Jennifer didn't recall any of her friends mentioning how challenging it was when they brought their babies home. It seemed like days since she'd had a shower and worn anything but pajamas. She was exhausted, frustrated, and annoyed with her husband, Matt. He never seemed to be around when she needed him.

The baby was nearly eight weeks old and nothing seemed to be getting any easier. Everything was hard. *Everything.* Breastfeeding was a nightmare. She'd seen three lactation consultants who had three different opinions as to why things were so difficult and painful. Their advice would help for a bit, raising her hopes, but then things would go back to the way they'd been. She could just as well be a cow for all the time she spent dealing with milk. Maybe it would make things better if she supplemented with formula—a thought that horrified her because good moms don't supplement. At least that's what she'd been telling herself.

Even worse, the baby didn't seem to be sleeping for more than two hours at a time. On top of that, her baby girl had decided the early morning hours were the best time to be hungry or—for goodness' sake—ravenous.

Jennifer had come to the conclusion that she just out and out sucked at being a mom. She was convinced that she deserved the award for Worst Mom of the Year.

Jennifer looked around from her position on the couch and took stock of her reality. For the first time, she saw what appeared to her to be flashing neon signs that now defined her life.

EVERY PLATE AND FORK IS DIRTY

The kitchen was an utter disaster. Dirty dishes everywhere. Food left out on the counter. Spaghetti sauce drying on the stovetop. When did it become so difficult to load a dishwasher or run a sponge over a surface? Just looking at it all made her exhausted. If she couldn't get to cleaning, why couldn't Matt at least try?

OH LOOK, DIRTY DIAPERS

Then there were the dirty baby clothes piled up in a corner of the living room. The smell of soiled diapers everywhere. If she'd turn her head, which she was too worn out to do, she'd spot the pile of damp towels on the bathroom floor. The mildew-stained shower curtain. The empty shampoo bottles spilling over the trashcan.

How did this become her house? She was used to being organized and putting things away when she was done with them. The problem was, Matt wasn't helping with anything.

I LOOK LIKE A DIRTY DIAPER

Who could blame him? She was a disaster. She couldn't remember the last time she brushed her teeth. And her hair? Well, she'd worn it in the same scrunched-up mess on top of her head for what seemed like weeks now. If she was lucky, she could manage to get out of her PJs by the time Matt got home from work. But who knew the last time she actually had clean clothes or something to wear other than sweats or stretched-out yoga pants?

NOT SHOWERING IS THE NEW BLACK

Not that it mattered, because she hadn't left the house for what felt like weeks. And her body was nothing like what it was before the baby. Her stomach sagged, her breasts were four sizes bigger, and not in a let's-put-on-a-cute-shirt-and-go-out kind of way, but rather in a they-won't-stop-leaking-and-they-freaking-hurt-and-all-my-shirts-are-stained way. Everyone had told her that she'd quickly drop the 30 pounds she'd put on during pregnancy, particularly if she breast-fed, but after eight weeks she still had 29 pounds to go. No doubt, Matt was disgusted with her.

ALL BABY AND NO PLAY MAKES JENNIFER A DULL GIRL

Jennifer was going stir-crazy to boot. The only friends she'd seen were the ones who occasionally dropped off food for her and Matt. But even that little mercy seemed to be coming to an end now that the baby was almost two months old. She was desperate for some adult connection. It was so hard to be away from work.

BOND, BABY BOND

Part of her thought that she wanted to be home with the baby, to spend those early months creating an unbreakable bond. She had made that clear and conscious choice. Both she and Matt had. But the fact was, all she did was hold and feed the baby 24/7. She just wanted a break so that she could go out and have coffee or lunch with her friends and not feel so completely braindead. She wanted to talk about something other than the best diapers to use, a milestone the baby was meeting, or the amount of sleep she was getting or rather not getting. She'd be happy to talk about who did what on a family vacation or what someone had purchased at Home Depot. Anything but baby talk.

Jennifer glanced at the TV. Her only company was a streaming episode of *Grey's Anatomy*, which played incessantly in the background. She wasn't sure if she could talk anymore to someone who'd say anything back. Sure, it was getting easier, what with the occasional smile she was starting to get from the baby in response to something she had said and yet it wasn't enough. A horrible thing to think, let alone say aloud.

She'd been so desperate for some kind of connection during those early weeks that she'd spent nearly every free moment—as brief and far between as those moments were—monitoring social media. But she vowed to stop scrolling Facebook and Instagram. She couldn't take seeing all her friends going out for happy hour looking bright-eyed, dressed to perfection, free. If they were too busy to come and visit, as they claimed, how were they able to go out evenings?

Did Matt even want to be around her? Hell no. He got to spend time at work five days a week. Talk to his colleagues and friends. Go out to lunch. Have human contact. Shower without interruption. Wear clean clothes and look fresh and engaged. In the morning, he'd give the baby and Jennifer a peck on the cheek and be on his merry way. It wasn't fair. She was always the one getting up through the night, feeding the baby, and changing diapers. Yes, they'd decided to take on these roles, to divvy up responsibilities the traditional way, but now Jennifer couldn't help thinking, rightly or wrongly, that their deal was unfair.

Jennifer knew that her growing resentment was doing them no good. But she couldn't seem to stop it. To add fuel to the fire, they had no time as a couple. As much as she loved knowing Matt was on his way home from work, the excitement didn't last long after he arrived. Five minutes wouldn't go by before the excitement turned to disappointment. It seemed like he always had something better to do than spend time with her. Before it got dark, he'd be off to mow the lawn, which had looked like shit for years. Now, all of a sudden, he was invested in taking care of it, as if a photographer from *House & Garden* were going to show up at any minute. She just wanted him to hold the baby for a while so that she could use the bathroom and actually brush her hair and teeth. Maybe sit with her in the evening, if only for half an hour, and munch on popcorn, watching TV together, the way they used to.

How had this little baby she'd wanted so much cause Matt to back away? Why was he not into the baby as much as she was? Why did he still get time for himself and she didn't? Why did he always seem to be watching TV on his own while she struggled to nurse and feed the baby?

MATT'S PERSPECTIVE

What the hell? When did Jennifer become so uptight? She's on me all the time. (And not in a good way!) All she does is bitch about how she's alone all day, how she doesn't get a chance to even shower or brush her teeth. The minute I come home, she's on my ass, wanting me to do something. But the second I pick up the baby, it's a frickin' constant critique; I don't hold the baby right. And even though I put a diaper on the baby, I didn't do that right either. She makes me not want to do anything. Honestly, it doesn't make sense for me to come home, to even want to come home, because I'm clearly not needed. Somehow she's decided I don't know how to wash dishes anymore, let alone change my own kid's diaper.

Matt is exhausted and overwhelmed and trying to balance helping out at home, where he always feels judged, with trying to perform at his job on just three hours of sleep. He's not doing very well and it is getting to him. Things are falling through the cracks on the job and he's sure everyone notices. (What a perfect time to get fired this would be.) He works through lunch trying to get things done so that he can go to the gym but he's way too tired to work out anyway. He hasn't had any social time with his colleagues or friends for weeks. Is he being selfish? He doesn't know because he's too exhausted to think.

All he wants to do is take a few minutes to decompress when he comes home, before he starts his second shift. But the looks he gets from Jennifer when he walks through the door could kill. And to think she gets to stay home with the baby while he's working overtime so that she can take the time off. She doesn't even appreciate it. Not only that, she somehow can't manage to do the dishes, let alone pick up the package from the post office like he'd asked her to do two weeks ago. And when he walks through the door, before he can get his coat off, he's handed the baby. Did she ask, "How was your day?" He didn't hear it if she did ask. Now he has to change a diaper in his work clothes. If the smell of poop permeated them, would he even know? All day at work he thinks he smells poopy diapers. He wonders if he's going to lose his sense of smell.

This wasn't how it was supposed to work. What happened to their deal?

Will I Ever Feel Like a Human Being Again?
I wish I could say that Jennifer and Matt's scenario was a rare one, but it's not. Truth be told, it's common. Even a professional therapist like me can get caught in the very same death spiral.

After I gave birth to our first child, I too was overwhelmed and exhausted. I doubted my competency, not only as a mom but also as a wife. It didn't take long for me to figure out that staying at home all day was not my thing. I needed to get out, go places, but as I mentioned in Chapter 5, I feared taking the baby outside the home. How would I manage his care on the run, in a different setting, when I barely managed in the comfort of my own home? What would people think of me if he cried? Where would I change his dirty diapers? And of course, how would I manage to breastfeed him in public? I could imagine the dirty looks that people would give me if I pulled out my boob in the back of a restaurant.

When my sense of isolation got bad enough, the research I did to find baby-friendly places to take my son was also important for me to find other mothers I could relate to and connect with. I started going to a local moms group and a postpartum workout class. They saved my sanity on so many levels. I felt like a real-live human being once again, not an automaton. I got to talk to other women, who could actually say something back to me, not just stare silently into my face or howl when I set them down.

You Mean, Other People Have Babies Too?

Some of the mothers in my group seemed to be having an even more difficult time than I was. They complained that their husbands came home late from work, ignored them but gushed over the baby for five minutes, and then moved on to do something for themselves. And here these women were, struggling with feeding and with their babies crying nonstop during the "witching hour," and there was no family close by to come over and help them out.

What happened to this being the most magical time of our lives? Maybe we've been cursed.

Misery Loves Company and Fresh Air

Thank goodness I wasn't the only one totally unprepared for what having a baby would do to me or my relationships, most of all the one I had with my husband. Stretching during my workout, doing my damnedest to touch my toes, I started mentally compiling a list of things I wish I would've known before I brought home my son.

This list became the foundation for the popular workshop I conduct with my husband, "Mine, Yours, Ours: Relationship Survival Guide to Baby's 1st Year." It was the experience that Rick brought to the workshop that made it all the more valuable. Because, although women typically signed up for the workshop and brought their partners along for the ride, it was the male perspective that allowed everyone to feel like they had a voice. It's easy to feel resentful when you don't understand the other partner's perspective.

Welcome to Les Misérables Workshop

The parents and parents-to-be who sign up for our workshop often tell us that they want to make sure they don't end up miserable like some of their friends. They want to make sure they keep the relationship solid and the communication lines open and flowing even when they are sleep deprived. They want to make sure the relationship that got them to this place to begin with continues. They also want to learn how to manage self-care with all the new chores and time sucks that get thrown into the mix. You don't have to look far to see parents who have never made the transition, who have let themselves, their homes, and their relationships completely go.

GET SUPPORT BEFORE IT'S TOO LATE

I've seen couples who have come into my office way too late, who have gone too long before getting the support they need. They're the ones overcome with resentment, anger, depression, anxiety, and distrust. They don't trust that their partners will be there for them when they say they will. They don't trust that their partners will do the things they say they'll do, when they say they'll do them.

They want their relationships to be stronger; they want to feel closer because this is their family. Unfortunately, most of the time they feel like they are barely treading water. And with each additional child, the gap grows wider, the water choppier.

They tell themselves that when their children are older, they'll have more time together. When they show up at my office, they're often expecting their second or third child without having sought out any help or guidance with their first.

These couples haven't been on a date for months or even years. Their interactions are confined to things that they need to do to keep their children alive and fail to include things that connected them in the first place and that would bring them closer together. They may be close in proximity, but they couldn't be farther apart emotionally. It never seems to get easier for these couples.

When we're in my office, the three of us know a couple of things: (1) Estranged couples often get divorced. (2) An ounce of prevention is worth a pound of cure.

What About a Pound of Prevention Instead?

This is your time to create the life you want, the childhood for your children you did not have. To build a strong foundation so that you can thrive in your relationship, even after your children are grown.

Of course, no couple is an island; we need other people in our lives as well. We can't raise a baby, at least not easily, without additional support, love, and care.

Navigating this transition period seems so much easier said than done. There are important elements to consider, starting with a clear understanding of the status quo before you bring baby home. The following steps will help you identify what you will need to do to get through the difficult times.

Enroll in Relationship Care 101

Keeping your relationship going strong, attending to each other's emotional needs with a baby in the mix, requires some attention to connection. When we're exhausted, being intimate and having sex are usually the last things new parents want to think about, especially breastfeeding moms. One of the most important actions to take is to openly acknowledge that things are different in your relationship and then to talk about how they are different.

Remember, I work with couples in my private practice. I've learned just how common it is for a new mom to feel uncomfortable in her post-pregnancy body and how common it is for a new dad to not want to put any pressure on her because he knows she has a lot going on. Neither of them is asking for sex, and neither feels like the other person wants to have sex with them. It doesn't take a therapist to recognize the setup for disappointment and resentment.

Make sure to let your partner know that you want to be intimate, that you want to feel physically close and connected, even if you don't have the bandwidth for sex at the moment. As contrived as this sounds, make plans for intimacy, even if you have to clear your schedule or put time for it on a calendar.

Intimacy doesn't have to mean sex, although sex is vital to a healthy relationship. Intimacy is about a loving, private connection between two people. The most common way for two people to get away from it all is to create a date night.

It seems that the list of reasons why or how we can't make time for each other is endless. And over the years, couples have shared unique and challenging reasons why spending time together is even more difficult when they have a baby. But the couples who are able to find a way to make time for their relationship report back to us that they feel so much more connected.

GET THAT CONNECTION BACK

For date night, consider:

- Game night
- Video games
- Table topic cards
- Wine and chat
- Foot massages
- Dinner without kids

Date night isn't the only way to regain connection. You can fit time for focusing on your relationship into other areas of your life. It doesn't have to involve hiring a babysitter and sitting across from each other in a restaurant.

Things to try:

- Work out together side by side at the gym or stroll around a museum and then go to dinner.

- There's nothing like picking up a new hobby together, especially if both partners are learning it at the same time; it means no one is the expert. Taking classes together can become successful bonding time.

- Try sneaking away for an occasional lunch together. A lunch date is a great way to reconnect and escape the drudgery of everyday responsibilities.

- Twice a year, schedule a weekend getaway, even if it means scrambling to find family members or others to watch the children.

- If you can't leave your home, make a point of planning a once-a-week dinner together after the kids are asleep.

- Form a babysitting cooperative. Find other families you'd trust to watch your kids and trade off babysitting while one couple goes out.

RECOGNIZE WHEN THE TIME IS RIGHT

You want to feel connected to your partner? You want to feel like having sex again, before the next ice age? Remember that all positive interactions are foreplay.

Here are just a few ways of getting a new mother interested in some action. (This, Dad, is mostly for you.)

- Give her a baby-free moment to finish her meal.
- Clear the table.
- Do the dishes.
- Give the baby a bath.
- Play with the baby.
- Allow her a few moments of uninterrupted time to just be.
- Tell her she looks beautiful after she's been up all night with the baby.

- Take the time to write a card or draft an email reminding her of the top five reasons that you love her.

- Give her a passionate kiss to spark the flame.

- You name it…

All count for a bit of something.

RICK'S TAKE

Catherine and I have been teaching our workshop, "Mine, Yours, Ours: Relationship Survival Guide to Baby's 1st Year," since 2010. While the information in Catherine's earlier version was great, the workshop was missing something. What it was missing was the perspective of the dad. It was missing, literally and figuratively, a male voice.

I believe that having a dad's perspective has made this a more meaningful workshop for the couples who have taken it. New dads get to hear that they are not alone, and new moms get to hear their partner's perspective. I also believe that it is good for new moms and new dads to hear from Catherine and I as a couple. New parents, hopefully, understand through our example that a strong relationship is possible.

There were many times early on as a dad where I felt like I was being helpful by mowing the lawn, finishing a home repair project, or something else Catherine saw as random. She would get super frustrated with me and snappish, but I didn't really understand. I thought I was actually being helpful and "getting things done." It just was not what Catherine felt was helpful or needed at the moment.

ENDNOTES

35 For divorced or separated couples: Though this list might need modification to your circumstances, I would argue that having a rock-solid, trusting, communicative, supportive relationship with your co-parent or main support person is just as important as it is for married couples. I will try to include tips for adjustments where applicable but consider this disclaimer permission to modify any of the suggestions in this book as needed to apply to your life.

36 Curt A. Sandman et al., "Prescient Human Fetuses Thrive," *Psychological Science* 23, no. 1 (December 2011): 93-100, https://doi.org/10.1177/0956797611422073.

37 Diana Divecha, "What Happens to Children When Parents Fight," Developmental Science, published April 30, 2014, accessed June 8 2020, https://www.developmentalscience.com/blog/2014/04/30/what-happens-to-children-when-parents-fight.

CHAPTER 9

Teamwork: There's No *I* in *Baby*

There's a famous phrase to promote teamwork: "There is no 'I' in 'team.'" There's no *I* in *baby* either. The point is, caring for a baby is all about teamwork. Everything you would do to ensure a successful joint operation in business, sports, or community applies to raising an infant. (Obviously, there is an *I* in *infant* but let's forget that for now.)

JILL AND STEPHANIE'S STORY
Jill and Stephanie had been together for three years when they brought their baby home. They prided themselves on the fact that they were well-prepared for their son. They had taken many steps to ensure that all would go smoothly. They had spent a lot of time prepping for the perfect birth. They had done all the research; they had visited the local hospitals and birth centers before opting for a home birth with a midwife and a doula. But following the baby's birth, they soon realized that they had done very little prepping for after his arrival. Jill was doing most of the childcare as she was breastfeeding around the clock, and Stephanie was taking care of "everything" else.

JILL'S PERSPECTIVE

Where is Stephanie? I've been sitting here all day with the baby, and I swear she's like a blur through the house. I miss spending time with her. Doesn't she know how lonely it is sitting here feeding the baby? Why doesn't she check in on us? I wish she'd come and hold the baby because I'd be happy to actually wash the dishes for a change. It feels like I never do anything but hold and feed the baby all day long.

STEPHANIE'S PERSPECTIVE

I'm not sure what to do with the baby. Jill has all the baby experience, having had younger siblings and babysitting her younger cousins, plus she's such a natural. Every time I hold him, he starts to cry. I dread the thought of being left alone with him.

Things became challenging as Jill felt like Stephanie was doing everything but spending time with her and the baby, and Stephanie felt like Jill had it all handled. Almost every interaction became snappish, and it felt like every comment was a criticism. It became very clear that each was more focused on what the other was not doing instead of on what she was doing.

Be sure to provide each other with support and encouragement. Having a new baby is a new experience for both of you. It can be challenging to have to try and figure out how to meet the needs of your precious new baby while also trying to manage all the other aspects of your life. It is important to be able to support each other and acknowledge how you are both in this together, as a team.

It is also important to acknowledge that each of you has your own strengths as a parent. You do not need to do things exactly the same way.

HONOR THAT EACH PERSON HAS THEIR ROLE IN THIS

Something I hear often from moms going back to work after maternity leave is that they continue to carry the brunt of the housework and parenting duties. But this is a fast track to burnout, to feeling overwhelmed and resentful toward your partner.

We have to keep in mind that while a parenting relationship is never perfectly 50-50, our needs are constantly shifting and changing. And we need to be ready to shift along with them. We have to be able to say to our partner, "This feels like too much," and ask them to step in and help.

This means letting them have their time and their tasks in helping with the baby. And letting them do things their own way. A concern we get from a lot of new parents is seeing their partner struggling. Your first inclination may be to scoop up the baby and say, "Let me do it." The problem with this is, it definitely is going to hurt the three of you in the end.

For one thing, it's squashing Dad's confidence. (And I'm going to use Dad because I'd estimate that in 95 percent of my experience, it is Dad.) It's also not letting him feel bonded with his baby. Second, you could be losing out on what could potentially be a break for you, which further drains your well. Third, if Dad isn't bonding with baby, that also means baby isn't bonding with Dad.

It's so much better to have two parents who are involved and supported than to have one who feels disconnected and one who feels overwhelmed, with them both resenting each other.

Ask For What You Want or Need

Sometimes I'll hear from parents that they get tired of having to ask their partner for help. After all, they have been together for years. How is it not as obvious to their partner as it is to them what needs to happen: "Why can't they just know what I need?"

I'll admit, I've felt that way before too. But the thing is, that line of thinking just isn't helpful. The reality is, your partner is not you. They do not live inside your head. They can't anticipate every little thing that you and the baby need without being told.

So you have two choices here: (1) You can decide that they should just know and see how that goes for you. (2) You can simply ask. And maybe you don't get what you want every single time, but I would put my money on your getting what you need much more often.

These tips are simple but implementing them isn't always easy. Still, it really is worth investing the time and energy. Doing the work little by little now and consistently throughout the years is much better than not doing the work and then trying to save a marriage later, when it might be too late.

RICK'S TAKE

As a brand-new dad, I felt that I needed to be ready to do anything and everything to care for our son. I was prepared to do all the chores around the house when he was a baby. What I did not plan for was actually asking Catherine what she needed and how she thought things should be handled.

Because I was not communicating with Catherine very well in those first few months, our relationship was not as strong as it could have been.

We got past this hurdle when we had our first date night as parents. That night we talked about how we wished we'd known how hard parenting would be before we brought our son home. This sparked an honest conversation about our expectations. It was during this conversation that I realized I had been doing what I thought was needed and was angry because my efforts seemed to go unappreciated. But I was doing what I thought was necessary without checking in with my partner to see what she needed.

After we had this conversation as a couple, we made a concerted effort to do a check-in at least once a day. This was a chance for each of us to say what we needed, what we expected, and how we could help each other.

CHAPTER 10

Talk, Talk, Talk; All We Do Is Never Talk

Communication will set you free or at least keep you from a lot of arguments. Here are some ways that couples have told us they make each day better.

Make time to check in with each other every day even if just for a few minutes. One of the biggest complaints we hear from couples is that they never communicate anymore. When you have children, it takes more effort to make time for each other. So get in a habit of taking 10 to 15 minutes each day to check in and find out how each other is doing.

> ➤ This is really just a quick meetup. It could take place 10 minutes over coffee before work or during the baby's naptime on the weekend.

> ➤ Here is where you touch base about upcoming events. Maybe you have a massive project at work, which could potentially keep you at the office later than usual. Maybe you suspect that the baby is teething so you know you're going to need to prioritize your own naps over doing the dishes or the laundry for the week. Or may-

be you need to prep the house because your mother is coming into town for the weekend. Whatever it is, lay it all out and ask for the help you need to get through it. This might be help that you need to outsource.

> A key part of your check-in is planning when each of you will take a break. Even if it's just a short break, carve out the space for it and hold that appointment with yourself as a sacred promise. This goes back to making sure that you're taking care of yourself. We have to help our partners do this too. Make sure you're coming through for your partner so that they can get the break they need too.

Every time a couple tells me that they are taking this advice and actually implementing it, they come back to me and say what a huge difference it's made. So just experiment with it and see if it works for you.

Acknowledge each other. Let each other know that you see what they are doing even if it seems small or you think they should be doing it differently. Be specific about how what they are doing is helpful. Often, Mom tends to be the one doing all the feeding and Dad the one doing other chores or household duties. Many mothers have complained that Dad seems to be absent when in actuality, Dad is trying to be helpful and involved. He is just doing the things that he knows how to do. Even if the lawn he is mowing is mostly weeds.

Be specific about what is helpful and what is not helpful to you. Do not assume your partner will know that it bugs you when they come home and chill in front of the TV right after work. Don't also assume what you are needing help with is obvious to anyone other than you. Speak up.

Instead of pointing out what the other person is or isn't doing, talk about what you are feeling. Instead of saying, "You always _____" or "You never _____," say "When this happens, I feel _____." This will completely shift the conversation away from criticism and defensiveness and toward understanding.

Ask, "How can we adjust? What can we do a little differently to help each other out?" There might be ways that you can reassign certain tasks to rebalance the workload. For example, maybe you ask that your partner gives you 30 minutes of free time before they chill in front of the TV. But doing things differently might not shift the workload at all. Sometimes solutions are as simple as daily check-ins with each other to see how things are going or to acknowledge each other's contributions with gratitude.

There are going to be rough patches in this parenting adventure. No doubt there will be times when one of you is doing the brunt of the work. One thing we parents learn very quickly, though, is that the work of parenthood is always changing. Nothing lasts forever. But with good communication and some understanding, your relationship with your partner will.

How to Communicate Postpartum
One of the biggest challenges we hear couples expressing postpartum is that they're just not feeling as connected to each other as they used to. This is partly due to being exhausted and overwhelmed by the onslaught of emotions, tasks, and fatigue that accompanies such a change. And it is also due to the fact that they've forgotten how to communicate with each other since the baby arrived. They have extensive conversations about the color and consistency of poop. They discuss with military precision the subject of diaper inventory control but hardly ever talk about other topics that revolve around raising their little one.

It's possible that because of their own upbringing, they never learned how to communicate under difficult circumstances or how to talk about difficult feelings without inserting resentment or blame into the conversation.

STOPPING TOXIC RESENTMENT

As silly as this may sound, we have to teach new parents how to communicate with each other. We have to teach them how to break destructive patterns of interacting, patterns they didn't freely choose but find themselves tied to anyway. Because when a new baby comes along, life will never be the same. If their toxic communication patterns persist, the resentment will lead to discord and will erect a wall between them. And the longer those patterns continue, the higher the wall will become and the harder it will be to tear down.

SHAYNA'S AND TYLER'S STORY

Shayna had just put the baby down to sleep, which, quite frankly, felt like a miracle. She figured she'd run to the kitchen to try and get dinner ready so that she could surprise Tyler when he got home from the gym. It had been ages since they'd eaten a decent meal, since they'd sat down together over anything that didn't require opening a box or heating up in the microwave. But the meal prep wasn't going smoothly, which was when Tyler walked in the door. The baby had already started crying in the other room and she hadn't even turned on the oven yet.

Shayna yelled for Tyler to get the baby and change the diaper. Seemingly in slow motion, Tyler took off his coat and put down his gym bag. Shayna wondered why it always seemed to take him such a long time to do anything she asked him to do. Couldn't he hear the baby screaming? Wasn't it bothering him too? Why didn't he want to take care of the baby, to keep the baby free of any distress whatsoever, as much as she did? What was wrong with him?

Shayna pulled open the door to the kitchen cabinet and grabbed a couple of dinner plates. She could still hear the baby crying in the other room. In fact, her breasts could feel the baby crying because she was leaking milk through her shirt. Slamming the plates on the counter, she stormed out of the kitchen after Tyler, only to find him doing some crazy thing or other in the baby's room. Sure enough, the baby still didn't have a diaper on. Tyler had her down on the changing table but he appeared to be doing everything but putting on her diaper. Shayna quickly intervened, showing him how to change a diaper properly. What she failed to notice was that the baby was perfectly happy, cooing in fact, delighted to be entertained by her dad. Tyler was doing it his way but to Shayna, it was the wrong way.

Shayna was frustrated and annoyed. She snapped at Tyler for what felt like the millionth time. Apparently, he'd had it with her once again getting upset for no good reason because he yelled back, "Fine, do it your way!" With that, he left Shayna alone in the room with the crying baby.

She quickly finished with the diapering, then pressed the baby to her chest in an attempt to soothe her. She didn't understand what was happening to them. Evenings used to be one of her favorite times of day. She and Tyler would reunite after a long day at work and make dinner together or go out and try one of the new trendy restaurants in town. Now it seemed that he was always off doing something in the garage. She wasn't sure what that "something" was since the garage always looked like a mess. It felt like their marriage was a mess too.

She missed talking to Tyler and laughing with him. Hell, she missed having friends, any friends to confide in. She could feel her fear bubbling to the surface. Where were things going? If she felt so alone now, if she and Tyler were fighting all the time, how would it be a month from now? A year? More?

Shayna was striving to care for the baby all on her own but only because she thought she was the expert at keeping the baby healthy, comfortable, and safe. She felt little sense of control over her life as a whole but in this arena she was the pro. She was used to being commended at work for doing a good job but she wasn't hearing praise at home from Tyler and that was causing her to question herself and her competency as a parent. Why did she think this would be easier?

Shayna couldn't talk to Tyler about her feelings, her concerns, her struggles, or her doubts, especially not now. She could hear the chainsaw starting up in the garage for the thousandth time that week. And even if Tyler were there, sitting at the table waiting for the dinner she'd struggled to prepare, they were both too tired to talk, to communicate with anything other than grunts.

SHAYNA'S PERSPECTIVE

I feel like I haven't stopped since my eyes popped open this morning at 5:30 and the baby needed to nurse, and then I scrambled to gather all my pumping supplies and throw a so-called lunch together before running off to work. I don't even remember if I kissed the baby before I left. It feels like the demands are nonstop. I had to pump, eat lunch, and answer emails simultaneously because it was the only time that I got to stop between meeting with clients and collaborating with co-workers. I'm so freaking jealous that Tyler gets to stay home with the baby. They seem so chill when I get home. But I don't even have time to change before Tyler heads off to the gym. He says it's so I get quality time with the baby, but I feel so frazzled. I just want a few minutes to settle in before he leaves. Because the baby seems to cry the whole time. Everyone tells me it's the "witching hour," but I can't help but think my baby hates me!

TYLER'S PERSPECTIVE

Being home with the baby all day is great, but it's such a long day. I can't wait until Shayna gets home so that I can have some downtime at the gym. I understand that she works all day but so do I. The only chance I get to feel like myself is that hour at the gym. The only bad part of going to the gym is knowing that when I get home, Shayna is going to start bitching at me the moment I walk in the door.

POSITIVE COMMUNICATION HABITS

Here's a short list of the habits I worked on with Shayna and Tyler to help them develop effective communication.

- **Listen.** This means you should *not* be formulating your response before the person speaking has finished what they have to say.

- **Keep it positive.** Avoid using negative words and phrases. Don't blame. For example, saying, "You always come home late and never think about us" sounds accusatory and can automatically result in a defensive response. Try saying, "I was feeling lonely today and have been looking forward to your coming home. So it made me sad that you were so late."

- **Make sure that your body language welcomes open communication.** Avoid crossing your arms, spreading your legs in a defensive posture, or frowning. Pay special attention to your facial expression.

- **When you have something important to say, avoid using a text or email to express it.** This often leads to miscommunication due to the inability to accurately convey tone and body language.

Tyler and Shayna took each day at a time putting these habits into practice the best they could. The suggestions also helped them come up with ideas to improve each other's day.

Remember, effective communication isn't always easy. When you're tired and overwhelmed, it often goes right out the window. So you have to plan for the inevitable and put a system in place to prevent your relationship from sliding into the ditch.

If you love your baby, which I know you do, you've got to be solid with your partner and that begins by keeping the lines of communication open. It begins by setting aside time to work on connecting. It's up to you to prevent the downfall of your relationship. And you can do that by following just a few basic guidelines.

WES AND JULIE'S STORY

Wes and Julie had been together for nine years when they had their daughter. They had met during their senior year in college, and after establishing their careers they spent time traveling, eating out, and meeting up with friends. While they spent lots of time together, they were both fiercely independent and had their own hobbies and ambitions. They were very supportive of each other's goals, often encouraging each other to take the next leap.

So when they welcomed their baby girl home, they were not expecting the impact it would have on their relationship. Julie struggled with "trying" to get Wes to do more to help with the baby, and Wes felt annoyed and frustrated with not being able to live up to Julie's expectations.

After months of what felt like totally ineffective parenting and partnering, they realized that they both were assuming a lot about what the other person would or should be doing. They realized that they couldn't do this parenting thing solo, but they hadn't had a conversation about what each of them could or would do. They needed to work together and actually talk to each other and not assume that the other person knew what was going on with them. They needed to acknowledge what each other was bringing to the table and find a way to support each other's needs and ambitions. And they needed to find a way to encourage each other where they were struggling.

These "rules" worked well for Wes and Julie:

Preventive rule 1: Make it a priority to talk with your partner on a daily basis, even if you have to schedule it on your calendar. And even if it's only for 10 to 15 minutes a day, take the time to check in.

Preventive rule 2: Find time to talk with limited interruption.

- Make a date to talk with your partner.
- Talk instead of watching TV.

- Walk 'n' Talk: Go for a walk together.

- Work together on household chores, e.g., making dinner together.

- Talk while in the car, traveling to activities.

Preventive rule 3: Come up with a list of questions that I promise you, you'll forget to ask. Check them off on a daily basis.

THE DAILY CHECK-IN WITH YOUR BEST FRIEND, YOUR PARTNER

Instead of just asking, "How was your day," pick a few questions that you can ask to find out a bit more about what went well and what didn't. This also can give you an opportunity to find out how your partner may need more support from you or others. Remember, these are questions you are both asking. Don't forget to take turns.

Questions to ask:

- What went well for you today?
- What was hard for you today?
- What is one thing that I can do to support you today?
- What do you need to do before you get home to help you shift gears?
- What do you need from me when I get home from work?
- What do you need when you get home?
- What do you miss most? How can we reintegrate that into our life?
- How are you feeling about being a mom/dad?
- What do you like about being a mom/dad?
- What hasn't worked and how can we fix it?
- What does your week look like? What do you need in order to accomplish those things?
- What do you need from me? I need _____ (cuddle, time, a break, etc.) from you.
- If you could have one thing this week, what would it be?
- Something we used to do on the weekend that I would like to try and do again is_____.
- What would you like to do for fun?
- I'm so appreciative when you _____ (help me with dinner, give me a break without my asking, wash the dishes, etc.).
- Three things I'm grateful for today are _____, _____, and _____.

RICK'S TAKE

Talking, really talking, and listening to each other is what got Catherine and I through our first child's first year. Finding the tools to communicate helped us stay connected as a couple. Without those tools and practices, we would have kept pissing each other off.

Sometimes we hear in our workshops that parents feel like some of the things Catherine has laid out here are selfish. New parents sometimes tell us that they feel like it is selfish to take time out for themselves or for their relationship. When we hear this, we always say ensuring your child(ren) have parents who honor and respect each other is not selfish. It is good parenting. Happy, connected parents are good, present parents. Keeping your relationship with your partner strong is something we do for our partner and ourselves, but it is also a gift we give our child.

CHAPTER 11

I Cried at the Hallmark Commercial

Now that you see there are ways to communicate and work together to make each other happy, here's something you may not realize can impact communication in a negative way. I call it the amygdala hijack.

The amygdala is the portion of your brain that is responsible for your emotions, survival instincts, and memories. Hormones and stress can trigger an amygdala hijack in ways that you may never have thought possible. Triggers include topics that when broached will send you straight through the roof.

If the topic needing to be discussed is too much to talk about now—meaning, you can feel your body respond with increased blood pressure, heart rate, and perspiration—your amygdala has been activated. You need to take time to cool down before continuing the conversation. Wait until you're both calm and capable of listening to what the other person has to say.

CALMING DOWN TAKES TIME
When you've lost your cool, blood pressure takes about 20 to 30

minutes to return to normal. Let your partner know that you need a time out. Take a break and agree to resume the conversation after that interim has passed. If it's still too difficult of a conversation to have right then, decide on a time to have it later. But make sure that you *do* have it. Avoid shoving a difficult conversation under the rug because it will resurface. I promise.

PREVENT AN AMYGDALA HIJACK IN THE FIRST PLACE

It's a good rule of thumb that if you don't like the way someone else is talking to you, do *not* respond to them in the same way or the conversation will go nowhere. You know the expression "Two wrongs don't make a right?" Well, two warring amygdalae do not make for a smooth conversation.

The amygdala is part of the limbic system, which is responsible for your emotional responses. An amygdala hijack can be triggered when we perceive that our needs are not going to be met. We go into fight or flight mode because we sense danger—in this case, danger that we are not going to get what we want from the person we depend upon. To keep from triggering an amygdala hijack, we have to first and foremost communicate our needs to our partner (or loved ones) in a clear and nonthreatening way.

Identify what each of you needs. This is important because needs are different than wants, which can seem frivolous to all involved. In this context, needs refer to practical as well as emotional support from your partner, friend, or parent. Most important, you can expect your needs to be different from those of your partner.

NEEDS CAN SET YOU OFF

To give you a better idea of what I mean by needs, here is a list of common needs you may not even be aware of. And you'll need to be aware of them before you can communicate them effectively.

- **Need for practical support.** Assistance in terms of help with chores around the house or with the baby, changing diapers, feeding the baby, holding the baby so that you can do self-care (bathing, sleeping, eating, exercise).

- **Need for emotional support.** Sympathy, empathy, or understanding, e.g., sitting with you, holding your hand, listening to you and not fixing anything or trying to make anything better except to ask, "How can I help you? Can we figure this out together?"

- **Need for sleep.** You need at least six-plus hours of consistent sleep daily or at least every other day. Importantly, you can never catch up on sleep, and sleep is mandatory to alleviate depressive symptoms. Not getting enough sleep can have a lot of negative health consequences and also can affect your judgment and your reaction to situations.

GET YOUR ZZZS

Dr. Michael H. Bonnet, a professor of neurology at Wright State University School of Medicine, suggests how you can find out how much sleep you need.[38]

Allow yourself to go to sleep at a reasonable hour and wake up on your own. Avoid all environmental factors, including the baby. Get whatever help you need to watch the baby so that you can find out what you need and do your best to get this much sleep daily. At least attempt to get this amount every other day so that your body can be rejuvenated and you can think clearly.

BASIC NEEDS TO REMEMBER

Positive relationships, which are improved by good communication, grow best when we have three things going for us:

1. **Enough regular sleep.** In the early days of bringing baby home, it seems that parents struggle to get two to three hours of uninterrupted sleep; it's just part of the game. But you can-

not go too long down this path or you will begin to fly off the handle, cry at the slightest provocation, and/or devolve into fighting with anyone who crosses your path, even when you really don't want to. Simply put, sleep is important for emotional health. It's very difficult to function effectively on minimal sleep for an extended period of time, so at the very least, try to stagger your and your partner's bedtimes so that each of you can get at least one five- to six-hour block of sleep per night.

2. **Good nutrition.** This means plenty of water and healthful meals with sufficient protein, fats, and complex carbs.

3. **Exercise.** Even if it's only for 10 minutes a day, three times a week. Any kind of movement that makes you feel good and you look forward to will improve your mood a thousandfold. Exercise could mean taking a walk around the block, dancing to your favorite tunes, following a YouTube workout video, or engaging in any activity you enjoy that gets you moving.

ENDNOTES

38   Denise Mann, "How Much Sleep Do You Really Need?" WebMD, published November 30, 2010, accessed June 8, 2020, https://www.webmd.com/sleep-disorders/news/20101130/how-much-sleep-do-you-really-need#1。

CHAPTER 12

How to Get 40 Winks or 20 Really Good Winks

If we had a dollar for every parent who told us how tired they were, we would have more than enough money for our kids' college savings and then some. The simple fact is that a new baby ensures you will not be getting enough sleep. (If you happen to have that rare baby who sleeps through the night from day one, no new, exhausted parent wants to hear it, so don't tell them. They probably will only wish you ill will.)

CHRIS AND KAREN'S STORY
Chris and Karen were struggling to get cumulative hours of sleep since their daughter arrived home four weeks prior. She seemed pretty chill during the day but the wee hours of the night were proving to be more difficult. They realized how much they were grappling with each other in regard to their communication and their connection.

KAREN'S PERSPECTIVE
I honestly thought that babies slept all the time. I didn't realize that you

actually had to read books about how to get your baby to sleep through the night or even hire sleep consultants. I know, I was so naive. And seriously, my easygoing, calm, cool, and collected husband is so damn snappish in the middle of the night. Oh my goodness, when he asks me, "Do you want me to get the baby?" I feel like he is setting me up. Yes, of course I want you to get the baby. I'm exhausted from what feels like marathon feeding, and I'm pretty sure that I haven't slept a full hour yet. But if I say I do, he is going to be so irritated with me.

CHRIS'S PERSPECTIVE
I feel like there is no good option for me when the baby cries at night. If I get up and the baby needs to be fed, I feel like I have just wasted my time because Karen has to breastfeed our daughter. But If I don't get up, Karen acts like I am not pulling my weight. There has to be a solution to this problem but I am honestly too tired to think about it or talk to Karen about it.

TAKE ANY AND ALL OPPORTUNITIES TO GET SOME SLEEP
Everything seems worse when you are not getting your sleep. We now know that new parents lose hundreds or even thousands of sleep hours in their child's first year. It can feel impossible to find opportunities to get some sleep, and it may even feel like you will never be rested again.

People tell you to sleep when the baby sleeps, though that can be difficult. Even if you can't fall asleep, we still advise you to lie down and rest. That means no electronics. Maybe a book or a magazine but something calming and restful.

Rick and I have heard over and over again about couples struggling with middle-of-the night sleep. In fact, it is one of the biggest struggles in those early months and sometimes throughout the first year and beyond. It was middle-of-the-night sleeplessness that was a catalyst for us to have a heart-to-heart conversation. It didn't happen in the middle of the night; that was not a good time for us to have a conversation—consider the amygdala hijack. But the following morning, we sat down and talked about our trouble getting through the day and the night.

Couples have told us that only one of them is getting up through the night because they are "not working yet," and their partner is, so they feel like they owe it to their partner to be the one who gets up. The challenge is that we all have limits to our mental well-being when we've had endless nights of little-to-no uninterrupted sleep. That is when we start to see more resentment in parents and their feeling like they never get a break. These partners report that they feel like everything is on them because they're not back at work yet or because they are exclusively breastfeeding.

It is important to start exploring alternatives. Every couple's situation is different and every baby's needs are different, but here are some ideas we've heard from couples that have benefited them in the sleep department.

- Trade off so that one partner gets baby until 2:00 a.m., the other after. (Be sure to consider who gets baby if baby starts crying at 1:58 a.m.)
- Alternate nights with who gets up.
- Bottle-feed at one point in the night so that Mom can get at least one good five- to six-hour block of sleep.
- Agree that one sleeps in on Saturday, the other on Sunday.
- Arrange for a friend or family member to spend the night and care for baby.
- Hire a night nanny for a couple nights a week.

Lack of sleep impacts our communication skills. Research shows: "Sleep disruption is associated with increased activity of the sympathetic nervous system and hypothalamic–pituitary–adrenal axis, metabolic effects, changes in circadian rhythms, and proinflammatory responses."[39]

In other words, our ability to respond to our body's fight or flight response is affected. Classic amygdala hijack.

ENDNOTES

39 Mann, "How Much Sleep Do You Really Need?"

CHAPTER 13

What to Expect When You Have Expectations

It is not uncommon for couples to share their frustrations because one of them has an idea about how things should go and their partner has completely different ideas. This was the case for Steve and Christie.

STEVE AND CHRISTIE'S STORY

Christie nags Steve about everything, or at least that is what it feels like to him. There are constant critiques about everything he does or doesn't do. She becomes annoyed when he doesn't respond to her, but he doesn't respond to her because he's learned to ignore her so that he doesn't blow up at her.

STEVE'S PERSPECTIVE

I would like to come home from work just once and not be given a laundry list of things to do. And when did Christie forget that I've been watching kids since I was 10 years old? I can change a diaper better than she can, and I could prove it if she'd let me. I wish she'd give me a chance to come in the door, change my clothes, and transi-

tion a bit before she launched into her list of chores. She totally doesn't get that I've been up to my eyeballs at work, and I haven't had five minutes to myself either. I'd be happy to play with the baby while she drinks a glass of wine and makes dinner. Seriously, that would be good for us all. She's so freaking unreasonable that I wish I'd gone out with the guys after work. I swore to God that I'd never feel this way about my wife and kid.

CHRISTIE'S PERSPECTIVE
I feel like I've gotten nothing done all day. But if we took at least 30 minutes when Steve got home, we could get so much done and then we could get on with our evening routine. I wish he could see how efficient we could be with our time, and when we got the baby down we could hang out together and catch up on one of our Netflix shows.

There's a lot out there telling us about what to expect as parents. We see these picture-perfect posts on social media and read articles about how life with baby should be. But the truth is, until the baby gets here, we really have no idea what's going to happen or how the changes will impact our family.

EVALUATE YOUR EXPECTATIONS
Sometimes what we expect to happen or dream of happening gets in the way of what really happens and makes us upset about what we are experiencing. Your baby will not do what you want them to do: Eat when and how you want them to and sleep how and when you want them to. But that can also be the beauty of parenting, because having children makes us grow in ways we never expected.

Having unrealistic expectations can be detrimental. They can cause a range of side effects such as anger, resentment, anxiety, depression, guilt, a sense of failure, difficulties in bonding with baby, and strain on your relationship with your partner.

If you want to feel like a failure, try setting the kind of goals that are impossible to meet. Then if you want further proof of your inadequacies, not just as a mother but also as a human being, try following your friends on Instagram and Facebook as they post their flawless photos and gush over their ruggedly handsome, loving husband and adorable, cheerful baby.

Notice how "magical" this time is for them, while you're wiping the spit up off your shoulder and realizing that you forgot to eat lunch (and breakfast). Their euphoria only serves to highlight your incompetence. If that doesn't make you wonder if you were ever cut out for parenthood, I don't know what will.

The problem is, when our expectations don't match our outcomes, we set ourselves up for either pleasant surprise or bitter disappointment (and possibly even trauma).

Remember that there are a lot of things changing all at once. Your status quo is anything but "quo."

HANNAH AND RUBIN'S STORY

Hannah had great plans for her maternity leave. She hadn't had more than a week's vacation since she and Rubin got married, and she'd been told that babies sleep all the time. Her expectations were on overload.

She was going to enjoy herself and be super productive. She'd reorganize the closets and assemble photo albums for the last five years. She couldn't wait to be able to work out every day so that she could get fit—and back into her pre-pregnancy jeans. Her friend Gina was back in her size 2 jeans just after her little one was born; she was going to do the very same thing. She figured she'd walk every morning and then hit the gym in the afternoon when Rubin got home. Or do a yoga video while the baby napped; she loved all those vinyasa sessions you could pull right off of YouTube. And there was a list of recipes she couldn't wait to try out. Maybe she'd try something fancy, like pheasant under glass or prepare an entire meal of raw foods. Also, there was that online course she finally would have the time to do and get the final credits she needed to complete her master's degree. She should have finished the degree three years ago but life had gotten in the way. Now that she was taking the extra time off from work, she might as well do something worthwhile with the downtime.

But unfortunately, this wasn't the case. Hannah was more tired than expected, and every time she would try to put the baby down, he'd start crying.

HANNAH'S PERSPECTIVE
What am I doing wrong? The baby is not sleeping even though I've read books on crying it out, the "gentle sleep" approach. Nothing seems to help. And on top of that, I'm not getting anything done. I'm going to go back to work having accomplished nothing.

Hannah's best-laid plans were overloading her emotional circuits. She became more and more frustrated, angry, and defeated. She figured that if Rubin would just leave work a little early, things would be so much easier for her. She could even run to the gym when he got home. After all, he was able to work out during his workday. He hadn't gained a ton of weight; he had time on his hands to look after his fitness and health. She knew that exercise would help energize her and increase the endorphins in her body and make her feel good. And she really needed those feel-good endorphins now. She needed to depend on her blood chemistry because the support and help she figured she'd have from her parents and her mother-in-law weren't working out in the way that she'd imagined.

RUBIN'S PERSPECTIVE
Hannah came into motherhood with a picture of how everything was supposed to be. Whenever I suggest that we need to dial back those expectations and accept the situation as it is and work to make it as good as possible, she has a meltdown. I wish I knew how to talk to her about this without it becoming a fight.

Hannah's expectations were the foundation for her current disappointment. Here's the deal: In the early weeks after bringing home a baby, your main job is to recover from delivery. All other expectations are ludicrous at best. You'll also be feeding the baby nonstop, often for hours at a time.

Now I wish we could say Hannah is a rare case but she's not. Especially when you have a Type A personality, it can be challenging to realize that things will not go according to plan.

Resist the Pressure to Jump Back into Things

I'm going to guide you through the minefield so that you can prepare for the changes brought on by a new baby and minimize the negative impact. To do this, we must first create realistic expectations of what will and won't be possible in those first few weeks of your baby's life. In other words, to get you headed in the right direction. To help you enjoy it, remember it fondly—in other words, to cherish it.

So What Can Really Get Done in a Day?

Nothing. Or at least that's what you should tell yourself. Then as you productively tear through the day and get a couple of things accomplished, you'll feel great. But tell yourself you'll get five things done, and you finish just two and you'll feel super frustrated.

Before we have a baby, we feel like we've got it together. We have a routine that works smoothly, a rhythm, and lots of predictability. For the most part, we consider ourselves pretty successful, accomplished even. We take simple things for granted. We get ready for the day, make breakfast, organize ourselves for work, perform in our job, meet with friends, have a relationship with our partner, and so on. We might gripe once in a while when things don't go our way, but for the most part our days flow smoothly.

Then after much anticipation and excitement, we bring this beautiful baby home. We expect the same level of success or ease.

We've been told that babies sleep a lot and to make plans accordingly. To just make sure to sleep when the baby sleeps. We're advised not to worry about the mess; there will be time to clean up when the baby is older. We decide, given this deceptive bit of information, that now is the time to finish our master's thesis, to remodel the kitchen, to move to a new house to accommodate our growing family.

And many new parents attempt one or several of these things. I mean how hard can it be? They will be home all day.

Except that it is hard. It's often described as one of the hardest transitions you will ever face. Just think about everything that changes dramatically, and all at once, and then ongoing, for years. You are learning about this new person, and they are demanding and show little-to-no appreciation at first. They give little feedback, and if they do, it seems like they're unhappy. You are thrown into situations you have never experienced before, and you have to learn new skills and better ways to communicate.

And now you want to take on another venture while the baby naps? The thing about a baby's napping in the first year as the baby grows is that it is most likely unpredictable. Remember, you will be tired and exhausted beyond anything you have ever experienced before.

CHAPTER 14

How to Know Who's Done What and How to Forget That Immediately

Kyle and Joanna had it up to here with each other. Both were self-employed and had some flexibility with their schedules but that didn't help. This was their first baby. How did their parents raise four and five kids, respectively, and not die from exhaustion? They felt like zombies for days because neither was getting any deep sleep. Kyle blamed any hallucinations on delirium from sleep deprivation. One night at 5:00 a.m. when he went to check on the baby, Kyle thought that he saw a pirate in the hallway. He hoped that he was hallucinating, or else he needed to buy a sword.

Kyle had always been so impressed with how bright-eyed Joanna was at 6:00 a.m. Joanna jokingly would describe to him what a sunrise looked like, since she was sure that he had never seen one. Kyle was a night owl, and no matter how much he tried to adjust so that he could be a morning person like Joanna, it never happened.

Here's where Kyle and Joanna say they couldn't believe they hadn't thought of the solution sooner. They decided to divide the night into two shifts. Anytime the baby woke up before 2:30 a.m., Kyle would handle it. Joanna took the early-morning shift. If they heard the baby cry, it took only a quick glance at the clock to determine whether it was their turn.

Suddenly, they were getting enough sleep for Kyle to stop seeing pirates and for Joanna to stop having to hear about his seeing pirates. As time went on and their son's sleeping habits changed, they would make adjustments to keep things fair. They felt so much better that they had so little stress about the baby's sleeping habits and that they could choose to disagree about other things.

Feeding, changing diapers, comforting, feeding, changing diapers, comforting— when you're living the movie *Groundhog Day*, suddenly it doesn't seem so funny. On top of that, all the things you have to do every day before baby don't just disappear. You can eat from paper plates and turn your dirty clothes inside out only for so long.

KEEP TRACK, NOT SCORE
Check our website, HappyWithBaby.com, to get some tools and worksheets to help you keep track of all your to-dos. Keeping track of who is doing what is important to make sure nothing is slipping through the cracks but that's as far as it goes. No keeping score!

If you've installed a scoreboard on the wall of your master bedroom that says, "Things I did" and "Things you think you did," you may want to try a different approach.

There is no fair way to evaluate who is doing more or who is doing it better. If you are feeling overwhelmed, talk with your partner. Chances are very high that they are feeling the same way.

READY FOR BABY WAKING UP THROUGH THE NIGHT?

The number one point of contention for couples may be how to handle the baby waking up through the night. This happens when both parents are working and even when one parent isn't working (well, not working outside the home anyway) and hasn't had a full night's sleep in days or weeks.

When my son was born, we didn't have any "plans." In fact, neither of us even remembers having any conversations about how we were going to deal with getting up in the middle of the night. We really didn't know what we were getting ourselves into or how it would impact the way we handled things.

When our son was about eight weeks old, it had been a particularly rough night, or maybe it was just that there had been several nights when it had felt like neither of us was getting any sleep. We both had been up at least once or maybe even several times feeding, changing our son's diaper, and trying to soothe him back to sleep, and we were exhausted, which definitely made us irritated with each other.

WE BOTH KNEW THE SCORE
Several times through the night, Rick was positive that he had gotten up the last time with the baby. He felt like he was doing more, changing diapers, finding pacifiers, getting me water to drink. However, I was positive that I had gotten up the last time and that I was doing more because I had to breastfeed, and it felt like each feeding took hours.

The thing is, we both were doing more throughout the day, and neither one of us was getting any quantity or quality of sleep. Neither one of us was in a very good position to keep score. And there's no real way to keep score when it comes to taking care of your child.

Does each thing you do count for one point? Or does breastfeeding count for more points than finding a pacifier? How many points is a diaper change, and if the diaper is poopy, does that count more than a wet diaper? Does your phone receive an alert every time your partner scores a point? Would that system cause more or less frustration and anger?

DISCUSSIONS LEAD TO SOLUTIONS OR AT LEAST UNDERSTANDING

We talked about our middle-of-the night problem the following day (because—go figure—at 2:00 a.m., we weren't able to effectively communicate or listen to each other), and we had a constructive conversation about what was not working for us during the late nights and early mornings.

Rick was able to express how he was feeling, and I shared how I felt. We were able to listen to each other's needs. Believe me, it wasn't necessarily that we agreed on each other's perspectives; at first our reasoning didn't make sense to each other. I thought he might have a head injury that I wasn't aware of. That's okay because we were talking and not being angry.

What did happen was that we were able to start trying to figure out how to make the nights easier or more manageable for both of us.

We were able to start having better conversations more regularly to try and avoid pitfalls. We thought about how we would do things differently so that we weren't so frustrated, resentful, and angry.

We were able to recognize that being parents was hard for both of us in different ways. This helped us to start identifying the signs that one of us was taking on more than the other or feeling overwhelmed.

Try to remember:

- The reality is that things probably aren't perfectly 50-50. They likely never will be for the rest of your parenting or married days. That's because things are always in flux, especially with a baby in the picture. One of you might be carrying the brunt right now, but that pendulum will swing and it will swing again and again.

- Noticing how your partner is contributing and helping (and thanking them for it!) will go a lot farther than dwelling on what they aren't doing.

- Ask for help. (If you haven't noticed yet, this is a recurring theme.) If you need a break or you're feeling resentment building up over all that you're doing, make a list of every single task and decide whether your partner or someone else can pick up the slack.

You may be asking yourself how in the world you can get some help at home when you're so exhausted that you can't even think of what to ask for.

It's a real struggle. There are so many things that demand our attention. So many things that need to get done. But, as important as we are, they *all* don't need to be done by us, do they?

No, of course not. But if we don't do all these things, who will?

Well, for one thing, the world won't fall apart if the dishes don't get done that night. So take care of you first, even if that's just fixing yourself a cup of tea or finally taking that hot shower you're overdue for. Then start working out a plan for how to better manage things for you and your family. Start by making lists of all the things—big and small—that need to be done. And take a few minutes to consider the following:

- What are the things that can be done only by you?

- What are the things that could lighten your load immediately if someone else would jump in to handle them?

- What are the things that are so overwhelming, you don't even know how to make them better or easier?

- Which tasks or problems are you willing to put money toward solving? Which tasks or problems are better solved by recruiting family members or offering a trade with a friend or automating with an online tool?

You can answer these questions more thoroughly by using my Postpartum Support Matrix worksheet, which you can download in the *Postpartum Planning Workbook* at HappyWithBaby.com. This gives you a place to hold all your to-dos, including the things that you do without even thinking because those tasks are part of your workload too! Besides keeping all your to-dos in one place, you can indicate who is performing which task when and how often, along with as much or little instruction as you want to provide. The worksheet also reveals which things you need extra support with so that you can begin delegating to friends or family or to paid support, like a nanny or a dry-cleaning pickup service, a meal delivery service, etc.

Not comfortable asking for help? You can post your list on your refrigerator and when visitors ask how they can help, you can suggest that they take a look and jump in on whatever task they like. (Because the boss doesn't do *everything*. They delegate.)

It's not uncommon to hear from moms in my private practice and our workshops that they feel so overwhelmed with the idea of asking for help, they don't even know where to start. They are used to doing everything for themselves and are really good at it too. They also struggle to ask because they see it as a sign of weakness or a failure on their part. This couldn't be farther from the truth. Asking for help is necessary because we only have so much capacity to do things.

Am I the Only One?

Are there things that *only you* can do? Sometimes they might be things that you're not willing to ask someone else to do either because you have your own system for doing them or because you love doing them. Or let's face it, sometimes it just doesn't feel right or comfortable to ask someone else. Of course, these reasons are all OK. But if you're feeling overloaded, you might want to consider relinquishing control on a few of them.

Start delegating. The tasks might seem small, like taking out the trash or wiping down the bathroom sink. But they can add up to making a big difference not only in your having to keep them in mind with all your other to-dos but also in your feeling supported and connected to others. Asking for help with these little things can help you get in practice for asking for help with bigger things, like doing laundry.

Find the best support options. Friends and family are good options to start with. But sometimes you can enlist technology. Be prepared for this to cost a bit of money. Do research or ask around for services to best assist you and your family. These can include online banking, meal planning, or even ordering diapers.

Troubleshoot challenges. Typically, these are the most difficult things to tackle or ask for help with but are the most important to work out. For example, if you are having a hard time breast-feeding, can you get support from La Leche League or a lactation consultant at your hospital, or maybe give yourself permission to use bottles? If you are recovering from a C-section or other birth trauma, what would help you to heal? If you're terrified of leaving the house with baby, can you ask a friend or your partner to come along? In many cases, a postpartum doula, therapist, or other professional can help with these things. If you're struggling with postpartum depression or anxiety, you obviously can't hand your PMAD over to someone else but you can seek support.

Also keep in mind that one person's "hardest thing ever" might be another person's "piece of cake" and vice versa. Try to resist passing judgment on yourself for struggling with something that seems so simple on paper or to other families. Use what *you* are feeling as your guide.

It Will Pass Faster than You Think
This "new baby" time is a short period in your child's life. You will be tired. You will feel overwhelmed. You will ask what the hell you

got yourself into. But this time doesn't last forever and things will get easier.

LET YOUR PARTNER FAIL

Each of you will have your own learning curve; some things will be easier for you and some will be easier for your partner. But it's important that both partners are given the space to come into their own as a parent.

LET YOUR PARTNER DO IT THEIR WAY

What we often see happening with new parents is that Mom wants Dad to help more with the baby and Dad wants to help more with the baby too. But then Mom will hear the baby crying and deem it a tortured cry and feel like she has to save the baby from Dad's clumsy ways. Or she will be watching Dad's every move and see him struggle with finding his own way to do something—or he just isn't doing it the same way she does—so she'll swoop in and take over, sometimes saying, "That's not how you do it!"

Resist every urge to do this.

Not only is it overburdening Mom to keep an eye on Dad but also it is crushing Dad's confidence as a parent. He needs to find his own way of doing things. His way may be very different from Mom's way but that's OK. In fact, it is better for baby to roll with different parenting styles than to need to be dressed or fed only one specific way. Because which is better: A mom who is overwhelmed, exhausted, and resentful and a dad who feels left out, frustrated, and confused? Or a mom who feels balanced, rested, and supported and a dad who feels competent, confident, and bonded with baby?

There will be things that Dad struggles with that Mom doesn't but the reverse is also true. That's the silver lining in the learning curve: You likely won't be struggling with the same thing at the same time so you can support each other. Besides, just when you think you've got stuff down, you can count on your baby to change stuff. There's no such thing as mastery here.

JAKE AND KELLY'S STORY

Jake and Kelly attended our workshop. Kelly admitted to us that she tended to be a Type A personality. She'd stop Jake in the middle of attempts at taking care of their baby's needs. Jake would become frustrated and self-conscious.

DID IT WORK?

I ran into Kelly several months later at a mom's group. She shared that Jake had been in the bedroom changing diapers and she could hear the baby crying. She wanted to go in and take over so badly. She knew that she could get the diapering done quickly and with minimal crying from the baby.

Kelly said she remembered our telling her to let Jake figure things out on his own and if he needed help, he could ask for it. If she was always going to the rescue and always correcting him and being critical, there was a good chance that he would stop helping her. Kelly also said it was probably the last time that she heard the baby crying when Jake changed the baby's diapers. The best part was that she was beginning to notice Jake's bond with the baby increasing as he started playing games like a peek-a-boo with the baby or dancing after diaper changes and the baby would giggle and laugh a lot.

This also is a good parenting reminder. When your children are learning to walk, they fall down. You may help them get back up but you don't decide to carry them forever. They get competent, and fast!

YOU DON'T NEED TO BE A "BABY PERSON"

It's fair to say not all of us are baby people. Some of us love the new-baby phase and some really struggle. But this doesn't mean that you love your baby less or that you're a bad parent. If you aren't a baby person, you might find that toddlerhood or middle childhood, starting when your little one enters kindergarten, is your favorite. It's probably natural that we do more when we're in a phase we love more. That's OK. The point is, you don't have to love every phase but there's always something in every phase to love.

CHAPTER 15

Five Strategies for Handling Unwanted Advice

You're going to hear a lot about parenting, especially from friends and family, who will claim to have perfected every nuance of child development. It may cross your mind that their children all had challenges, like eating their toys. This will not stop them from giving you advice.

Take everything you hear from those around you with a grain of salt. They typically mean well but sometimes things that your family and friends say can be upsetting and hurtful. Maybe it's because you're tired and already doubting yourself but just because someone recommends something does not mean that it is the right thing for you.

Nevertheless, how do you deal with parents who raised their child perfectly 30 years ago? For example: "Our baby slept on his stomach and we survived."

Really, the bar is that you "survived?"

Or what about the neighbor who says you're a bad mother if you watch television in front of your baby or feed them formula or anything else that she didn't do?

It never fails—the most well-intentioned parents, relatives, friends, and even random strangers all seem to have something to say about what we are doing as new parents. And sure, when we are well-rested and secure in ourselves and our abilities, we can handle these statements with ease and grace, but it's all the other times that get us off-track. Sometimes way off-track.

It doesn't hurt to put together a little script that you and your partner have ready to go. Talk through with your partner how to respond when these situations arise. (I can assure you, they eventually do. If I had a dollar for every piece of unsolicited parenting advice that I've received from complete strangers...) That way, you're not stumped for how to respond, you know that you and your partner are on the same page, and the risk of saying something regrettable is dramatically reduced. It's best if your script has a positive ring to it.

Think "buddy" cop movies:

- "Did we ask your opinion, punk?"
- "Let's take this guy out back and beat the crap out of him."
- "We're sick of talking to filth like you, so now we're judge, jury, and executioner."

OK, this list does sound fun. But you can maintain a united front and still be pleasant about it.

MIKE AND TINA'S STORY

Mike's mother had a reputation for being very intrusive and she also happened to be a nurse. This meant that she seemed to have all the answers or at least she thought she did. Tina was feeling apprehensive about having her around. She also felt like Mike was going along with whatever his mom had to say. It all felt pretty judgmental, and he let it go on and on and never backed Tina up. It became even more difficult because Tina was already feeling inadequate.

We discussed how important it was to have a united front. To back each other up in those moments when Mike and Tina were making choices together as a couple.

THIS IS HOW WE WANT TO DO IT

In our workshop, we've heard from many couples who have the dreaded family experts: the pediatrician father, the neonatal intensive care nurse aunt, the sister-in-law who's been a nanny since she was 13 years old, you name it.

No matter who suggests an alternative to whatever they think you're doing wrong, the answer that both of you give is, "This is how we want to do it." Not "I'm doing it this way for my wife [or my partner]." Again, "This is how we want to do it." (If you still want to feel like a "buddy" cop movie, you can throw in the word "punk" at the end.)

Because Mike and Tina presented a united front and weren't wishy-washy about it, Mike's mother finally backed off a bit. Tina felt supported by Mike, which made their relationship a lot better and also made it easier for her to want to be around her mother-in-law.

It turned out that Mike's mom didn't even realize she was being hurtful and judgmental. She thought that she was being helpful. Still, that doesn't change the response (say it with me now): "This is how we want to do it."

THE AWARD FOR BEST SCRIPT GOES TO...

We usually have a couple come up with variations of scripts and use responses like:

- "Well, this is the way we want it."
- "This is the way we're going to try it."
- "We're going to try this way for a while, and we'll remember that tip for later if we need it."

- "I'm going to talk to my partner, and we'll think about it."
- "Our pediatrician recommended 'xyz' so we're going to try that out first."

If you're being pressured about anything, whether it's about what and how your child is eating or sleeping or even whether you're coming over for the holidays, there's always, "We haven't talked about that yet. So I'll have to talk to my partner and we'll get back to you."

Finally, end with, "Thank you for your suggestion."

Part III:
Taking Care of Baby

CHAPTER 16

Bonding with Baby

I almost didn't write this chapter. You already can find lots of amazing books out there about all the ways that you can connect with your baby. In fact, when Rick and I meet couples in our workshops, they usually have a pretty good idea of how they want to parent—whether they change their minds about *how* they are going to do that is another story.

But I decided that if the topic isn't addressed, it can be hard to answer the third question: "What are you going to do to make sure you bond with your baby?"

Sometimes people question why I made this the third question. Shouldn't bonding with baby be your most important aspiration? Of course it should. We are talking about *your* baby, your precious child. However, the first two questions are the ones that are most forgotten. The ones that get put on the back burner because you feel like you can't do all the things you need to do.

It's important for you to know that you can do all those things. Sometimes you'll be better at it than others. And sometimes you won't be able to do things in as much depth as you would like. The point I want to make is that you shouldn't focus solely on your child at the expense of yourself and your relationship. Your child won't turn out better because of it. And you and your relationship definitely will not turn out better because of it.

So what's the answer? How *can* you incorporate it all? First, don't look at bonding with your baby as something separate from everything else. You can incorporate the baby in a lot of what you are already doing in your daily life. Bonding does not have to be a separate task. Bonding is what you are doing with your child all the time.

- Find a task that you are going to do—washing dishes, dusting, picking up toys—and talk to your baby. Simply talk to them about what you're doing. Research shows that how you talk with your child can alter their brain.[40] As they get older, they will respond to you with babble and eventually words. These back-and-forth conversations increase your child's brain development and language skills. More important than the words you say is the tone you use when talking, with pleasant, comforting tones being the very best. Plus, these conversations teach your child about relationships and interactions with others.

- You can use opportunities like diaper changes, bath time, or story time. (It's *never* too early to start reading to your child.)

- You can even find ways to play with your little one. Yes, you can play with a baby! Maybe you mimic their coos and gurgles. Maybe you move their arms and legs around gently so that they dance a bit. Or you can strap the baby into a baby carrier and dance around yourself. Simply narrating your activities to baby builds the bonding experience.

It's OK in the beginning for this to feel weird or ridiculous or like you don't know what the heck you're doing. Just discover the style and techniques that work for you.

BECKY AND JEFF'S STORY

Becky and Jeff were excited to bring home their new baby. They had talked a lot about how they wanted to parent. They'd spent time with friends who already had kids, and they'd witnessed things that they *didn't* want to do. They felt pretty confident that things would go smoothly. Until they didn't.

BECKY'S PERSPECTIVE

I wish Jeff would be gentler with the baby. He's always throwing him up in the air and tossing him around. I don't think he should be doing this before the baby is a year old. What about his poor little head? Jeff gets frustrated with me when I ask him to stop. I always feel like I'm telling him what to do and what not to do. This is not the egalitarian marriage that I thought we had.

JEFF'S PERSPECTIVE

All of a sudden, Becky is dictating everything. Even though we talked about these things before, now it seems like she wishes I would just sit and hold the baby while I looked at stuff on my phone. We talked about a friend who did this and said we wanted to be more engaged. I am, and it seems too much for her to handle.

Each parent is trying to figure out how to be with their baby. We even know of one dad who drew a mustache on his baby's face when his partner wasn't looking. At the time, his partner wasn't thrilled (I promise you that the baby was not harmed in any way), but she said she was able to laugh about it later and realize that it was his way of figuring out how to be himself around his new baby.

I'm not necessarily encouraging you to start doodling on your child but hopefully you get what I mean: don't take things so seriously and always be yourself!

Moms, realize that dads are not going to do it the same way you do. Do not hover over them and criticize. Let them get in their groove. Many dads have told Rick and me that they never feel like they do things right when moms hover or get critical. As a result, they stop participating. No one wants that to happen.

Consider the science behind play: Research shows that dads play with their children in very different ways than moms do. Moms might play gentle, cognitive games with their children, while dads tend to play more viscerally and physically. These different modes of interaction teach children how to regulate their emotions in intense situations and also build trust and a sense of independence.[41]

We each have a unique role to play in parenting. It's important to encourage each other and to let each other figure out how to be the best parent to your child. Make sure that in your quest to have a healthy and happy baby, you're not adding more pressure on yourself.

ENDNOTES

40   Sophie Hardach, "How you talk to your child changes their brain," World Economic Forum, published February 28, 2018, accessed June 8, 2020, https://www.weforum.org/agenda/2018/02/how-you-talk-to-your-child-changes-their-brain/.

41   Jessica Michaelson, "The Progressive Dad's Dilemma," The Gottman Institute, published March 24, 2014, accessed June 8, 2020, https://www.gottman.com/blog/featured-blogger-dr-jessica-michaelson/.

CHAPTER 17

Developing a Community of Sidekick Support

You can't do this alone. It's not a sign of weakness if you ask for help. More important, you shouldn't have to do it alone. We are supposed to have a community of support.

As we talked about being a Batmom and meeting with your "sidekicks," maybe you realized that you don't have a support group to ask for help. You thought, "No one could ever care for my baby as well as I do."

Many new parents tell us that they feel way too overprotective to allow anyone else to care for their baby; no one can do it as well as they can. This is absolutely right. No one can care for your child as well as you can. But if you don't take care of yourself by getting a breather, you won't have your best self to give to your child. This is where developing a community, a group of trusted people who will do a pretty good job, is key. Not only will you get time off for yourself—some space to be with your partner, some precious downtime—but your baby will reap the socializing benefits as well.

It is so important to make sure that you are getting time for yourself and your relationship. Babies who grow up around arguments, tension, and violence may experience developmental delays and/or adverse health consequences. Studies show us that maintaining a strong, healthy relationship with your partner is good for you and good for your baby.[42]

If there's one thing that will make a mom do something, it's finding out how it will help her child. And when you spend time away "filling your cup," not only will your baby be excited to see you again but also you will be refreshed and able to be present with your baby. Win-win.

Look, some people have a hard time asking for help; it's simply not in their nature. They don't see the signs that they are meandering and moaning like a cast member of *The Walking Dead*. You should be an energized and positive person around your child, not someone who looks like their appendages could fall off.

For some reason, many of us have decided that we should do everything on our own; we're used to being superhuman. Supermom does everything on her own, right down to making baby food from scratch, reading to her baby, and hugging the baby every 30 seconds. Since you believe you're Supermom, you resist all offers of help. You can do it all on your own—after all, you're Supermom.

I'm here to tell you that you don't come from the planet Krypton and it's OK to say yes to a helping hand, to have someone do something for you. If someone asks how they can help you, that means they want to make your life easier, if only for a while. Why on earth would you not take them up on it? When, as I will say again, you are from Earth, not Krypton.

WHAT IF NO ONE IS OFFERING YOU HELP?
Maybe you've moved to a new city or your friends and family are crazy-busy or have forgotten what it's like to have an infant at

home. If you don't have a good support system in place, it's very important to find one or to create one for your little family.

First, reach out to your family or friends and let them know that you're doing well but you're up to your eyeballs in diapers. Tell them that you need to go out for a short time and ask if they could watch the baby. Explain that you'll have everything ready and it'll only be for a short time. After the second or third time you reach out and still don't receive their help, be honest and let them know that you are overwhelmed and would really benefit from a helping hand.

If you have no family or friends around to help or the family or friends you do have are not helpful, another way to get support is to find a community through a local parent meetup, church affiliation, or library's story time group. Don't be afraid to ask questions, exchange phone numbers, or set up a time to meet for a play date or a moms' night out. Fellow parents everywhere will appreciate your stepping up to the plate and making things happen.

My experience tells me that if you're struggling to find a community, there are others in your area who are struggling to find one too. Look online. Meetup (meetup.com) is a good place to browse different groups of parents or moms or even dads who are looking for support systems or playgroups.

With Meetup, you can find groups who have common interests, like yoga for families, coffee klatches, regular playgroups, etc. If you have a community resource webpage for your area, look there too. If newsletters still exist at the time of reading this, check them out.

If you can't find an established group, create one yourself. A Meetup group that I started in 2014 has been such a great experience for the moms involved. Many of them have shared that they'd known no one locally for support and now they've found their best friend. What a thrill to be able to facilitate new connections.

Where else can you find people just like you? First of all, you've got to get yourself out of the house.

"BABY FRIENDLY" THINGS TO DO EVERY DAY TO HELP GET OUT OF THE HOUSE

- Moms groups (Check your local hospital for good support groups)
- Exercise classes where you can bring baby
- Music classes
- Child-friendly museums
- Library story time (Some even offer times specifically for babies.)
- Meetups (Check meetup.com for local parent groups in your area or start your own.)
- Playgroups outside your home
- Neighborhood park
- Walks to a neighborhood park or mall (Often the big department stores have nice changing/nursing stations)
- Lunch/coffee/walk with a friend
- Lunch with your partner at a restaurant or (as takeout) at their workplace

---

It might seem like such a small thing but it's critical to have that extra support in whatever form feels right for you. Whatever you're comfortable with will work out great. And what works for someone else may not work for you; know that's OK.

We aren't meant to do this alone. Reach out for help. Accept a hand. Make space for fun and connection—whatever it takes to get that support and stability you need.

> **BONUS TIP:** Parenthood is a much better place to be when you're not there all by yourself.

SEEK GUIDANCE AND SUPPORT

Build a community. This is especially crucial if you don't have a family support system locally. (And make sure you connect with parents who have enjoyed being a parent.)

List five to 10 people you can call in a pinch. Seek out parents who have older children, even by a few years, to offer encouragement.

Some options:

- Neighbors
- Parents' friends
- Coworkers
- Hospital support group (Usually the facilitator who leads is a good resource)
- Moms groups
- Meetup groups
- Congregants at your place of worship

Attend a workshop, with or without your partner, that normalizes what being a new parent is like. This might be "Mine, Your, Ours: Relationship Survival Guide to Baby's 1st Year";[43] The Gottman Institute's "Bringing Home Baby";[44] or a workshop by Becoming Us.[45] Or check your local hospital for listings.

Let's get real: It's one thing to find emotional support, to have a community that feeds you and your baby; it's another thing entirely to hand over your infant to another caregiver. That's the part that freaks us out the most. But from personal and professional experience, we know the importance of finding someone to give you a break, for yourself and as a couple.

ENDNOTES

42 Annamarya Scaccia, "Self-care isn't just good for moms—it helps protect your kids, too," Motherly, accessed June 8, 2020, https://www.mother.ly/life/taking-care-of-ourselves-can-protect-our-children-from-inheriting-toxic-stress.

43 "Our Workshops for Parents," Happy With Baby, accessed June 8, 2020. https://happywithbaby.com/classes.

44 "New Parent Workshops," The Gottman Institute, accessed June 8, 2020. https://www.gottman.com/parents/new-parents-workshop/.

45 "Professional Live Events," Becoming Us Family, accessed June 8, 2020. https://becomingusfamily.com/professional-live-events.

CHAPTER 18

Your Personal Mary Poppins

The fear of leaving your newborn with some else is a real concern for many new parents. It can be a bit reassuring if you have family members who live close by and offer to help. But unfortunately, the care and support we thought we would have does not always work out the way we had hoped.

EMILY AND BRANDON'S STORY

Emily and Brandon had assumed their parents would be available to take care of their son so that they could run out to the grocery store or even go on date nights. Unfortunately, things weren't working out that well. Brandon's parents were older and Emily didn't feel secure about letting them watch the baby on their own. Emily's mother was suffering from carpal tunnel syndrome so she didn't want her mother carrying the baby around the house. She wasn't even sure that her mother would be able to change the baby's diapers.

EMILY'S PERSPECTIVE

It is so frustrating that we don't have more help. Our parents are willing but not really able. It seems like all my other friends with babies have help. I don't feel comfortable with anyone but Brandon watching the baby.

BRANDON'S PERSPECTIVE

I thought that we would have help. I realize that our parents are older but I think they could at least watch the baby while we're home and we could take a nap or even get some things done around the house. I know that Emily's friends have offered to watch the baby so I wish she was more comfortable with saying yes.

Emily and Brandon are not alone when it comes to not having adequate help. We hear from couples all of the time that do not get the help from their parents they thought they would, for many different reasons: They still work, they travel, they have health concerns, the relationship with them is toxic. Whatever the reason, it can be upsetting when we as new parents realize that our support system is not as supportive as we imagined in our pregnancy days.

Some parents tell us that they have their partner, who's supportive, but your partner is not a postpartum plan and is not an adequate support system. They need help and support, too, and you can only do so much on your own as a couple. So what are you going to do?

Okay, you've put it off for a while but you've decided to find someone who can give you a break for a date night, a shopping trip, or just a well-deserved breather. It can be difficult to let someone else care for your child but we really do need to take time for ourselves. There's no way around it, not if you want to stay sane and have a real relationship with your partner. We give so much to our little babies, especially in the early days, that it can be very hard on us because we're always giving and not getting much back.

Over the years, many couples have shared that they are afraid to leave their child with somebody else or that they don't want to because they feel like they're already gone so much during the day because of work. They worry that their child already spends too much time apart from them in daycare or with a nanny. We've had couples tell us that it has been five or six years since they went out on a date and that they're feeling disconnected from each other and even like they're just business partners or coworkers at home.

START WITH DADDY

The first step in mom's releasing her death grip (!) from her baby is to let her partner watch the baby. Contrary to popular belief, Dad is perfectly capable of changing diapers, soothing a tummy ache or sore gums, or giving baby a bottle.

Dad is more than capable of taking care of baby. It might not be how Mom takes care of baby but that is perfectly fine. It is actually good for the baby to have different caretakers. Different is not bad.

More important, the more that Dad is involved from the beginning, the more confident and more comfortable he will be in caring for baby—which will lead to a more equal divvying up of parenting roles and increase Dad's attachment to the child as well.

For those control freaks out there, start with a very short break. Maybe take a bath or extra-long shower. For the more daring, go for a walk or even a trip to the grocery store. Did you ever imagine that would be so much fun?

Mom especially needs to equip the trusted individual—in this case, Dad—to feel safe leaving the child with him. If you act like it's no big deal, then he'll embrace his competency. If you act like it's the end of the world, well, he's going to approach the baby like he's defusing a bomb. And that's not good for anyone.

FIND SOMEONE OUTSIDE THE FAMILY

This is where things get serious. Like Jennifer from Chapter 8, many a mom has to return to work. Most workplaces are not going to embrace your bringing your infant to work. Which means you're going to need to find regular childcare. Maybe you and your husband care for your child in shifts (if so, see Chapter 14: How to Know Who's Done What and How to Forget That Immediately). But more likely, you'll need to secure an outside source.

One of the biggest challenges for moms when they return to work is the guilt.[46] Whether you're reluctant to go back or glad, guilt will be your co-pilot either way. To offset some of this guilt, you'll need to trust that you've secured the very best person to care for your child.

How Do We Pick a Childcare Provider?

Take the time to pick a provider so that you feel confident your child is in the best possible hands. Have any potential provider come over and watch your child for a period of time while you're home doing household chores.

Not everyone is meant to be a childcare provider. You likely won't be hiring a 12-year-old or your grouchy first cousin.

So what do you look for in a provider? Think about which things are most important to you and your partner and what you want for your family. The qualities that you may identify now may be different in six months, a year, or even three years from now. They also might change as you add members to your family. Your list likely will vary from your friends' or your sister-in-law's. Remember, that's perfectly OK. Your family is unique. There's no one right answer to the question about which qualities you choose.

Qualities to Look For in a Childcare Provider
- Caring
- Nurturing
- Reliable
- Provides good references
- Knows what to do in an emergency (CPR trained, etc.)
- Has ___ years of experience (Be realistic)

QUESTIONS TO ASK A POTENTIAL CHILDCARE PROVIDER
- What hours are you available?
- Are you flexible if we're running late?
- Do you have three to five references who will vouch for your childcare experience?
- Are you trained in CPR?
- Which age level(s) are you comfortable caring for?
- What activities do you like to do with children? (Have them describe a typical day caring for a child to get a sense of how they interact and what they do. Ask for specifics, e.g., if they say they go to a park, ask what they do at the park: Do they push the child in the swing? Do they make up games to play? You want to get a sense of their ability to interact with a child.)
- Are you available to help with household chores during nap times? (What chores would you want them to do? Show them a list.)
- How would you handle a fussy child?
- What happens if my child falls down/gets hurt and won't stop crying/screaming?
- What would you do if my child won't go down for a nap?
- What would you do if my child won't take a bottle/eat?
- How would you respond to my child if they were not listening to you? (Get a sense of their reactions when dealing with something minor, like your child won't put toys away, and with a safety concern, like your child won't stay on the sidewalk when walking to the park.)
- What would you do if there was a safety concern and you couldn't get ahold of me? (You are looking for them to say they hope there is a list of other people they can contact, like another parent, grandparents, a friend, a neighbor, etc.)

While you go through the interview process, keep an eye out for qualities that you should avoid. If the relationship with your childcare provider is rocky during the interview process, it isn't going to get better with the complexities of taking care of your child.

Qualities to Avoid in a Childcare Provider
- Tired when arrive at the interview
- Cancels at last moment
- Overreacts to little things
- Glued to cellphone
- Will invite friends over or meet friends while on outings
- Knows everything and cannot take feedback

Finding a childcare provider is not a matter of if but when. At any stage of parenting, if you haven't gotten help from a provider, now's the time. Both of you deserve a little time to yourselves so that you can be the best possible parents for your child.

Finding adequate childcare is important for a multitude of reasons: To be sure you get self-care, to be consistent about setting aside time to spend with your partner, to be able to go to work. And all are reasons why it will be easier for you to better care for your child.

ENDNOTES

46   Ilsa Cohen, "The Anatomy of Working Mom Guilt," Working Mother, published May 17, 2010, accessed June 8, 2020, https://www.workingmother. com/2010/5/home/anatomy-working-mother-guilt.

CHAPTER 19

The Final Word on Everything You Need to be Happy with Baby

Here's the question that everybody asks: "How do we get back to the place we were, particularly as a couple, before the baby came, although with some modifications?" Well, that's what this book has been about.

Here's the hardest lesson to learn: The baby isn't the center of your world but only part of your world. (You may have just gasped but it's true.) Babies enhance your life and make it fuller in ways that you never thought possible and yet they can't take over every aspect of your life. It's not good for them; it's not good for you.

You've got to create a secure bond with your child and also foster their growth and development. If you're attentive to your child's needs while encouraging them to develop their independence and safely explore and master their world with your support, you are on the right track.

Flexibility and a willingness to grow and change are important. Because you're not just parents, you're partners. You're human beings with needs and desires. You have to figure out how to make all these pieces fit once a baby comes along, and sometimes these pieces have rough edges.

The trick is to set realistic expectations from the get-go about what's to come. Make sure that you get the help you'll need because we all need help from time to time. Establish a community and find a mentor to guide you when the road gets rough. And it will get rough.

THREE CRITICAL QUESTIONS

If you can always remember to answer the following three (familiar) questions throughout your child's lifetime, you'll keep yourself on the right track, come what may:

- What are you doing to take care of yourself? (What are you doing to feel good about yourself? What are you doing for you?)

- What are you doing to make sure that you're connecting with your partner? (Have you set aside time every day to check in? Are you going out weekly for a child-free date?)

- What are you doing to make sure that you're bonding with your baby? (Do you have a routine with them? Do you spend quality time with them?)

This exercise gets you thinking about how you'll nurture your three most important relationships. (Be sure to download your own worksheet at HappyWithBaby.com.) Don't underestimate the power of this exercise based on its simplicity! It gets right to the heart of your family's foundation. Brainstorm ways you'll nurture connection to yourself, your partner, and your baby. If you think of your family like a layer cake, this is how you'll make sure the entire cake is sweet. The cake can look messy or lopsided but if the sweetness is there, that's what really matters!

These questions may seem obvious, but did you ask them today or yesterday? And how did you answer? Some days you'll answer with ease and other days it'll feel next to impossible. Remember to communicate with your partner about what's working for you and what's not. You're a team and you need each other to make parenting and partnering work. Your child also needs you to be together to do this well.

You can be among the 30 percent of people who say their relationship wasn't damaged in their child's first year.[47] You have all the tools you need to be a Batmom or Batdad. Not only will you have children who will be a source of pride but also you will have a marriage or relationship that will be the envy of others.

As they say, "The days are long but the years are short."

Things to remember:

- The concept of "easier" comes with a caveat: I'm not sure that parenting ever gets easier. It's just that what's hard changes shape.

- Sooner than later you will again get a full night's sleep on a consistent basis.

- You will regain a social life.

- Your workouts will extend from lasting 15 minutes to again taking an hour.

- Your stifled desire for your partner will rekindle.

- You will start to recognize yourself, even if you discover that facets are configured in a new way.

- There's no coasting in parenthood! You'll gradually trade in your sleepless nights and poopy diapers for parent-teacher conferences and heart-to-hearts about bullying.

So that's it. Go have your baby (or enjoy your baby) and know that when you use the tools we have provided here, you can and will have a strong healthy relationship with your partner.

ENDNOTES

47 Shapiro et al., "Effects on Marriage of a Psycho-Communicative-Educational Intervention With Couples Undergoing the Transition to Parenthood, Evaluation at 1-Year Post Intervention."

ACKNOWLEDGEMENTS

I want to acknowledge and thank everyone who has believed in me and helped me through the process of writing this book. As with having a child, the birth of a book is not something we can do alone. I am deeply grateful for not having to walk alone on this journey.

To each of you who encouraged me to lean into my passion, to teach workshops, to speak to people, and to then formulate it all into a book - thank you. To those that edited and re-edit my words and who helped me find my voice to exactly the words I needed - thank you. To my wonderful friends and colleagues that continue to encourage me and believe in what I have to share - thank you. To my the clients who walk through the door and trust me with their stories - thank you. And to the brave couples who join our workshops, who are eager to deepen their relationship with their partners and children - thank you for continuing to trust and to teach us.

And last but not least to my family - for enduring the countless hours of hearing me talk about this book, watching me write it, and cry when things were overwhelming, but always did so in a loving and encouraging way - thank you and I love you!

CPSIA information can be obtained
at www.ICGtesting.com
Printed in the USA
LVHW030748271120
672639LV00006B/470